Praise for *Beyond Schizophrenia*

"Susie Dunham's heroic, heart-rending story in *Beyond Schizophrenia* is a beacon of light in the darkness of insanity. It shows that recovery is hard-won but possible for people who develop schizophrenia, despite a media that sensationalizes them, a society that shuns them, and a dysfunctional mental healthcare system that fails them miserably. All American Mike is more than "a perfect son." He's a shining example of success for 3 million Americans who suffer in silence."

—Patrick Tracey, author of *Stalking Irish Madness: Searching for the Roots of My Family's Schizophrenia*

"Every person in a leadership position needs to take the time to read this moving story of triumph over adversity."

—State Representative John Adams, Ohio House Minority Whip

"The fact that Michael bravely fought this disease, picked up the pieces and moved beyond it, should give others hope that one day schizophrenia will be seen as a treatable disease with no stigma attached."

—Sharon Goldberg, News & Reviews Editor, "NYC Voices": A Journal for Mental Health Advocacy

"*Beyond Schizophrenia: Michael's Journey* is a book that I couldn't put down. The story of Michael's parents Susie and Mark who support their son both in good times and bad really touched me. I really like the way the symptoms of schizophrenia are explained clearly. *Beyond Schizophrenia: Michael's Journey* is a must read."

—Bill MacPhee, Founder/CEO of SZ Magazine

"Susie Dunham holds nothing back. She is so refreshingly honest and personal that I found myself wanting to give her and every family member a big hug through their tears of courage."
—Larry Hayes, author of *Mental Illness and Your Town: 37 Ways to Help and Heal*

"This is a powerful memoir that captures the struggles many families encounter in helping a loved one with mental illness. Susan Frances Dunham's deep devotion to and support of her son are inspiring."
—Michael J. Fitzpatrick, Executive Director, National Alliance on Mental Illness (NAMI)

Cover art by Gary Wittenmyer
Author photo by Theo Dunham (Video Creations)
Cover design by Michal Šplho (www.michalsplho.sk)

Library of Congress Cataloging-in-Publication Data

Dunham, Susan Frances, 1954-
  Beyond schizophrenia : Michael's journey / Susan Frances
Dunham, Michael Dunham.
      p. cm. -- (Reflections of America series)
  Includes bibliographical references and index.
  ISBN-13: 978-1-61599-058-0 (hardcover : alk. paper)
  ISBN-10: 1-61599-058-5 (hardcover : alk. paper)
  ISBN-13: 978-1-61599-035-1 (pbk. : alk. paper)
  ISBN-10: 1-61599-035-6 (pbk. : alk. paper)
  1. Dunham, Michael--Mental health. 2. Dunham, Susan Frances,
1954- 3. Schizophrenics--Ohio--Biography. 4. Parents of mentally
ill children--Ohio--Biography. I. Title.
  RC514.D863 2011
  616.89'80092--dc22
  [B]
                                        2010032755

Distributed by Ingram, New Leaf Distributing, Bertram's Books
(UK), Hachette Livre (FR), Angus & Robertson (AU).

Modern History Press, is an imprint of
Loving Healing Press
5145 Pontiac Trail
Ann Arbor, MI 48105

www.ModernHistoryPress.com
Tollfree 888-761-6268   Fax: 734-663-6861

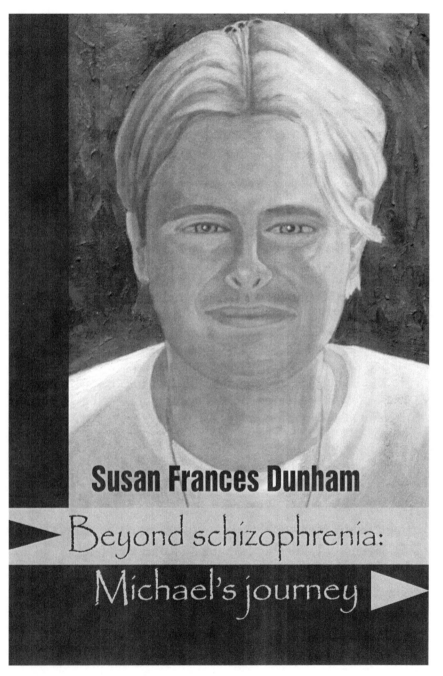

Susan Frances Dunham

Beyond schizophrenia:

Michael's journey

Reflections of America Series

Modern History Press

Contents

Foreword

Even if you haven't had a child with a mental illness, you'll find yourself cheering Susie Dunham as she struggles to help her son Michael triumph over his disability.

Yes, I've been there with my own son John – through a son's self-doubt; through the voices in his head; through his suicide attempts; through the struggles to stay in school; through the false starts at a job. But I know as Susie so painfully discovered: There is help for those with mental illness. There's hope. Indeed, there can be triumph over tragedy. That's Susie's story.

Beyond Schizophrenia: Michael's Journey deserves to be widely read. Its insights into a dysfunctional mental health system recount an all too-familiar experience for families who struggle to cope with a child's emerging mental illness. In that respect alone, the book stands as a compelling indictment and a call to action.

Much to her credit, from the time Michael is first diagnosed when he's heading back to college and a career in acting, Susie Dunham never loses faith. She's a retired nurse who knows well how to care for other people. But Michael is her greatest challenge, even from the time he's a sensitive boy through the hospitalizations and those inevitable letdowns. As regularly as the setting of the sun, a dark curtain seems to draw close on those rare moments of promise. She and her husband Mark remain undaunted. Susie's unwavering faith inspires other family members to enlist in Michael's great battle.

She holds nothing back. She is so refreshingly honest and personal that I found myself wanting to give her and every family member a big hug through their tears of courage.

You can read textbooks and the scour the diagnostic manual, the DSM-IV. You can interview psychiatrists and therapists. But few things will give you a clearer understanding of mental illness as Susie's powerful story. Read it for the storms in the life of this family. Read it for what it teaches about character, about love. Then read this story to watch as the clouds in Michael's life slowly but surely disappear.

—Larry Hayes, author
Mental Illness and Your Town: 37 Ways to Help and Heal

Acknowledgments

This book is dedicated to Michael Francis Ralph. He is my brother, my hero, my friend in need, my keeper, and proved to be the closest person to my own mother, in her absentia. Mike saved our family in every conceivable way.

My very personal thanks go to my best friend, husband, and soul-mate, Mark. You were always right next to me. Somehow, we understood each other right from the start.

Nancy Dunham, my mother-in-law, friend, and former teacher, deserves my deepest gratitude for her unconditional help as a developmental editor.

My dear friend, Monica Heineman, graciously donated her time and skills as a professional copyeditor. Thank you, Monica! Your generosity is known to many.

Sincere appreciation is extended to Gary Wittenmyer – artist, brother-in-law, friend, and uncle to Mike – for his oil portrait of Michael, featured on the cover.

May God bless Pam McGlothlin, for her tireless efforts to provide hope, support and education to people suffering from brain disorders, their families, and the community, as a leader in National Alliance on Mental Illness (NAMI).

My final thanks go to Victor Volkman for believing in the value of my story, and gently guiding me to its completion.

Prologue

It wasn't until after two years of writing short vignettes, out of pain and catharsis, when I believed that I actually might have started to write a book. Then, I realized what I had been trying to accomplish from the beginning. I wanted to put a beautiful face that belonged to a brave, kind spirit, on a catastrophic, horrific disease. I wanted to explain quite visually: this is what schizophrenia really looks like. It is a tragic disease that doesn't discriminate between the wealthy and the poor. Regardless of race, religion, or national origin, the disease is not a rare occurrence; however, it remains poorly understood.

Michael's journey as a healthy, "All-American" kid to psychosis, and back again, is depicted through my eyes and voice, as his mother and a former nurse. My training as a nurse, to use my five senses, allowed me to document what I saw, heard, smelled, etc. But, it was my mother's instinct to write how I felt about our experiences as a family. Schizophrenia may not always present itself exactly the same way, but usually occurs in a person's late teens to early twenties. The sadness of this untimely presentation is that this is exactly the period during which young people begin to thrive and grow as young adults.

If there is possibly some universal message that my book might bring to others, it certainly isn't exclusive to schizophrenia but to all parents who must face a frightening and life-threatening diagnosis in their child. My advice would be that schizophrenia is purely and simply an organ disease. When kidney functions are compromised, dialysis is the treatment. Failure of the pancreas to produce insulin results in diabetes, controlled with insulin given by injection. The list of treatments for dysfunctions of body organs is almost endless. Unfortunately, when the "Master Organ" of the body is compromised, because of chemical imbalances, stigma and ignorance prevail.

If it could have been possible to define the major goal of my writing over the last five years, the answer would have been resoundingly clear: Try to reach the parents of children who have been recently diagnosed with any type of brain disorder. No matter what they were witnessing, and no matter what suffering their child was enduring, recovery was possible.

Part I – Foreshadowing Events

Chapter 1 – "I Dreamed I Was a Broken Boy"

Many of the books that I read advised that it was a bad idea to bring babies or children into the parental bed to sleep at night. Babies need to find ways to comfort themselves to sleep and to gain their own independence in the world. Years later, I read that the practice of children sleeping with their parents was far more common than most parents would admit. Many mammals sleep with their offspring for years, including bears and other wild animals. Most likely, this instinct and practice is for the preservation of their young. In our case, it was for our own self-preservation.

Mike had developed itchy allergic eczema, asthma, and nasal allergies in rapid succession. Upper respiratory infections presented a continuous battle, along with simply coping with all of Mike's allergic symptoms on a day-to-day basis. Those early years were tough on all of us for many reasons. Mark and I quickly learned that we both had to hold down decent jobs to pay the bills so that we could provide a decent lifestyle for our little boy. We understood the harsh reality of life. Our employers really didn't care if our child was sick on any given day. They expected us to find a solution and show up for work! I confessed to my mother that we had Mike in the bed with us at night to survive.

"If you keep this up," she said, as kindly advice, "You'll never get him out of your bed." *I am certain that she had some first-hand knowledge of this, as she and my father had raised eight kids*, I thought.

By four months, Mike developed "Atopic Dermatitis," commonly known as allergic eczema. This problem escalated and became severe by the time that he was twelve months old. We tenderly bathed him in hypoallergenic soaps, later bath oils, applied topical steroids and administered antihistamines as prescribed by his dermatologist. We cut his fingernails short so that he could do less damage with his scratching, but often he dug so hard that he had taken the top layer of skin off his ankles, face, hands, behind his knees, and the inside of his arms at the bend of the elbows. Mike's scratching was so severe that he often actively bled because his digging at the itchiness went so deep. We tried putting him in footed sleepers, thinking that it would be harder for him to get to his ankles which were the main sources of his aggravated itching. He quickly learned how to un-zip them. We tried food elimination diets and nothing helped. The skin on his fingers and ears was extremely itchy and dry, remaining cracked and open for at least nine months of the year. Summers often brought relief; but even in adulthood, winters triggered the eczema.

"Please Mikey, try not to dig," we begged.

"I have to dig," was his childhood response, as we re-applied the topical steroids to his skin and gave another dose of antihistamines. During peak allergy seasons, spring and fall, Mike rubbed his itchy eyes until his eyelids were raw and stripped of the top layer of skin. As they healed, they always looked scabby. His crying and frustration, as he frantically scratched at the already open wounds, was painful to watch.

The asthma began when Mike was only nine months, but the doctors didn't diagnose it until he was over two years old. "Babies wheeze," was what I was told as we admitted him to the hospital, at eighteen months, in acute respiratory distress. Mike wasn't just wheezing, but grunting as he tried to get some air. His tiny ribs retracted with each labored effort. We were there with Mike in the hospital for hours. Finally, I told Mark to go home and get some sleep because he had to be at school the next day. I realized that things had taken a turn for the worse when they took Mike from my arms into another room to perform an arterial blood gas test. I knew what they were doing to my baby as I heard him scream. They had inserted a large needle into his femoral artery, at the groin, to determine how much oxygen was in his blood. The resident doctor returned shortly and told me that he might have to start IV steroids on Mike to stop the inflammation in his lungs.

"Tell me now doctor, is our baby going to make it? I just sent my husband home to get some rest. Should I call him back?"

He hesitated and looked very troubled. "I don't know yet," was his response.

This was simply the first of many episodes, with all of them equally awful and terrifying. Those early years were filled with trips to the emergency room to open up Mike's lungs. Mike's blue lips, loud wheezing, and rib-retraction as he struggled for breath always heralded a day spent in panic, or another sleepless night. Mike grew up with an aerosol mask attached to his face, delivering relief and life-saving medicine.

The next cruel version of "The Asthma Triad" announced itself as nasal allergies. Mike's nose ran constantly. His eyes were extremely puffy and his sinuses, inflamed because of allergens, were easy targets for infection. Once his sinuses were infected, the infection dripped down the back of his throat and inflamed his bronchial tubes, which in turn triggered his asthma. Infections became the worst culprits. One problem played off the other. It seemed that there was no winning this battle. There were specialists for all three problems. The dermatologist told us what to do about his eczema. The allergist had advice about Mike's asthma. The newly hired Ear, Nose, and Throat doctor wanted to put tubes into Mike's ears, but couldn't because we could not get Mike's asthma stabilized sufficiently to risk a general anesthetic. Sometimes the three specialists did not agree on treatment. Still, the appointments needed to be kept. Some-how, Mark and I kept those appointments, went to work, paid for private day-care, and kept Mike at the center of our lives. What a juggling act it was!

The list of allergens that triggered all three of these problems was endless. Cats, dogs, other fur-bearing animals, weeds, pollens, molds, and foods were triggers, along with infections. Mark and I fought the good fight together, but there was always a new mystery to solve, and we tried to solve the latest, one day at a time.

"If your kid has a snotty nose," we advised friends and family, "don't bring him around." Few listened. "If you have a dog, cat, or a fur-bearing animal in your house, we can't go there." Few understood. Often, a riddle presented itself unexpectedly.

One day, when Mike was five years old, he came home with a purple stain around his mouth. Immediately, I thought that another kind parent in the neighborhood had given him a frozen grape popsicle. Our refrigerator and freezer were always open to the other children. If we were having lunch, we invited Mike's friends to eat with us. If Mike got a treat, we offered the same to his buddies. Perhaps another mother on the block was returning the kindness.

Two more times, the purple stain around Mike's mouth was noticed. The second time, Mike had slightly swollen lips. We only understood this in retrospect. The third time, Mike's lips became huge and grossly swollen.

"Mike, your lips are swollen. What did you eat? Who gave you food, and what?" Mike finally remembered that for the last three days, he had been eating mulberries from a bush behind the neighbors' property. "Never eat them again, Mike," we said, as we gave him Benadryl and called his allergist. This was just another day in our lives. Mulberries were clearly a new trigger to avoid. We were grateful that his throat didn't swell shut and cut off his breathing.

Later, we tried allergy shots on two occasions. We could not complete the first round because of Mike's recurrent infections and fevers. The second round was almost completed when Mike was fourteen years old. When the first injections of the highest dose were administered in both of Mike's arms, the results were immediate and frightening. I had never seen an anaphylactic reaction in my many years of nursing, but then witnessed one. Mike developed huge hives on each arm at the injection site, had trouble breathing, and then swallowing, in rapid succession. The end result was another trip to the emergency room, with life-saving drugs given by the emergency room doctor, monitored by his allergist. We decided we'd have no more of this stuff. The risk outweighed the benefits. We'd maintain the avoidance of allergens rather than introducing them.

I look back on those years and wonder how we survived them. Mark was teaching full-time, coaching tennis for his high school, and attending graduate school in the summers. I was trying to advance my own career, one step at a time. The center of our small world was always Mike. We found ourselves not just parents, but nurses, detectives, and guardians against the awful world of allergies and infections. We never had enough money, time, or sleep. Together, we weathered the bottle feedings, diaper changing, teething, toilet training, and day care issues, along with the heartache of Mike's continuous symptoms. When we couldn't relieve his itching, stop his wheezing or wipe his nose without causing pain, which was always red and raw, he cried. In fact, he cried a lot. Sometimes, we cried right along with him. Our struggle wasn't just difficult. It seemingly went on and on forever, with only a few splendid moments of relief. Yet, it was nothing compared to what was to come down the road. Looking back, this was, frankly, just "boot camp."

In spite of all these daily troubles, our lives were indeed filled with joy. Mike was a resilient little guy, born with a sunny disposition. We thought that he belonged to us, but the truth was that he owned both of us right from the start. We were totally smitten with his broad smile and crinkled up, mirthful, and sparkly eyes. Even as a baby and a very young child, we could see the kindness, sensitivity, and intelligence that exuded from him. We never spoke "baby-talk" to him, not just because we thought that it wasn't the right thing to do, but because he deserved better. He seemed to understand everything that was going on around him, far beyond his years.

From infancy on, we tried all of the advised "sleepy time rituals." Rocking, reading stories, playing soft music, and slow dancing with our child in arms were just a few measures taken to promote a good night's sleep for all of us. We put Mike into his crib or "big boy bed," tucked him in, and hoped for the best. In the usual event that he woke up crying because of his scratching, difficulty breathing, or was simply sick, we knew what to do. We took care of the immediate problem with medication and put him between us, in our bed. When he felt comforted, he scratched and wheezed much less. We could hear him more quickly if there was a problem, and catch a few precious hours of sleep before the next grueling day.

One significant evening such as this stands out in all of our minds. We lovingly tucked Mike into his twin bed with "Brown Bear," his name for his brown-furred teddy bear. Mike had many bears and all of them had their own special names. He couldn't have been more than four and a half years old at the time, as he drifted peacefully asleep, with his arm around his second oldest and favorite teddy bear. Mark and I virtually caved in, falling into an almost comatose sleep the minute we crawled into our bed. For at least four blissful hours, we had achieved deep, restful, peaceful sleep that for once had gone uninterrupted. It must have been one o'clock in the morning when our four-and-a-half-year-old came shrieking and screaming into our bedroom. He pranced around like a marionette puppet controlled by invisible strings.

"Mom, Dad, I had a terrible dream! I dreamed I was a broken boy. I didn't have any head, hands, or feet, and I walked like this." We both sat straight up in bed and watched in dumb awe as we tried to get our wits about us. This scene was too painful to contemplate. How could a little boy like Mike have such a terrible dream? Mark slept closest to the door and easily hoisted Mike's "light as a feather" little body into the middle of our heavily quilted king-sized bed with his strong, young arm. Instinctively, I had raised the quilts in advance. We both wrapped our arms around our sweet little boy and tried to comfort him.

"This was just a bad dream, Mike," his father offered over and over, as Mike shivered in fear. Mark stroked his head and patted his back.

"Mike, we'll never let anything bad happen to you. Dad and I will always be there. I promise." After much talk about bad dreams and constant reassurances, the three of us fell asleep in an exhausted embrace, but none of us ever forgot that night.

Some things are so horrible that you could never "dream" of them in advance. These things are absolutely inconceivable, unthinkable. We have control over many things in life. For those things, we must take full responsibility to avoid calamity. Tragedy or an unhappy fate is self described and unavoidable. Mark and I convincingly made promises to our only child on that night that we couldn't keep. Years later, Mike became a broken boy.

Chapter 2 – When Did This Start?

Any parent who has witnessed the tortures of schizophrenia will ask themselves the following questions:

"Why didn't I see what was coming?"

"What were the warning signals?"

"What could I have done to stop this from happening?"

"What could I have done to protect my baby?"

The clues and answers only became understood after the disease had fully manifested, but they had indeed been there for a while. I had seen changes, but they were insidious and confusing. I had asked many questions, but the answers I received seemed logical. I thought that something was not right, but also believed that nothing was terribly wrong. The knowledge that I received by attending NAMI's "Family to Family" program, two years later, convinced me that Michael had exhibited many "classic" onset symptoms. His early symptoms were:

- Anxious moods
- Change in sleep patterns
- Weight loss
- Withdrawal, decline in function, and lack of attention to personal hygiene
- Illogical thinking and lack of insight

There is always a "Prodromal Stage" in schizophrenia. A *prodrome* is a symptom indicative of an approaching disease. For example, in the disease of measles, a person will first have sensitivity to light before the rash and other symptoms appear. I saw the changes, but confused most of them with the side-effects of caffeine and medications or normal conflicts that occur in young people's lives.

In the summer of 2004, Mike attended college in order to graduate on time. Mark and I understood that courses weren't always offered at the most convenient times, so we had to be prepared. Mark helped Mike to map out his plan for graduation, and Mike's summer session resulted in very good grades. Mike had changed colleges and majors since his freshman year, so this had put him somewhat behind schedule. Mark and I both thought it was OK that Mike didn't work that summer because we were financially prepared to cover the bills.

"Take your classes and go out on the boat this summer," we both told him. "You'll never get the chance again to have this freedom. Once you are in the work force, your employer owns you!" August came and we packed Mike off to live with his steady group of college friends and roommates. Life was good. We had a plan.

Cell phones have made the lives of parents much easier. We could call Mike at any time, just to see how his day was going. I tried not to call too often and seem the over-protective mother, but made myself readily available. Mike seemed happy, enjoying his 20-year-old, somewhat adult life in college. He was having fun and getting good grades at the same time. We were a contented and optimistic family albeit our separation.

Mike grew his beautiful blonde hair quite long that fall.

"Will long hair affect the way your professors treat you, in light of the fact that you are studying business?" I asked.

"No, Mom, you'd be surprised. They are pretty liberal about things like that here." Once again, I thought, *why shouldn't he grow his hair long now? He'll never get the chance again.*

Mid-October came, along with an upper respiratory infection that sent Mike to the college clinic. We met for lunch, mostly to reassure me that Mike's asthma was completely under control. As we stood at the counter of the local Big Boy restaurant to pay the bill, I was approached by a woman roughly my own age, in her fifties. Her whole purpose was to tell me that her eighty-year-old mother thought that my son was the most handsome man she had ever seen. "Mom loves your son's long hair!" she said. Of course I was flattered, thought it was funny, and decided that this new phase of long hair wasn't that bad after all, if an old lady could comment on it.

Our lunch at the restaurant involved all of my usual questions. "How are things going? Are you happy? Are you getting enough to eat? Do you have enough money?" All of my questions had been answered affirmatively. I drove home happily, remembering our conversation.

"Mom, the most unusual thing happened to me in one of my business classes. We had to role-play on video, and it was my job to solve a problem with a client. I barely looked at the script and ad-libbed the whole thing! My professor gave me an A and told me that either I was going to be the best sales manager in the world, or that I missed my calling and should have been an actor. I want to be an actor, Mom. You know that I always have." It was all true. From the time that Mike was little, he had been a performer, dancing around and imitating celebrities. This was no surprise to me, but we lived in the Midwest, not exactly a hub for screen acting. We had taken advantage of local opportunities for children to pursue personal interests, including cub scouts and music lessons, but acting lessons seemed out of reach.

"Mike, finish your degree and go someplace where you can pursue your dreams. Go there with a real and legitimate job so that you don't have to live in poverty." He was indeed beautiful, smart, funny, kind, and motivated. There was nothing that he couldn't do if he put his mind to it. Nothing that he told me was even mildly delusional; he was simply stating what he had always wanted, once again.

I know for certain that Mike was totally intact for all of the first semester of his junior year in college. His roommates later agreed with me after Mike's break from reality in the summer of 2005. Mike was engaging and enjoying life. He was intuitive about math and became popular as a tutor for anyone who needed assistance with their math courses. He had learned complicated tricks to solve problems from his father and as time went on, he could solve math problems without the use of a calculator. Sometimes, his teachers would count off points because he didn't show his work. He had solved most of the problem in his head and, quite frankly, was too lazy to write out the tedious steps.

Mike told me about the college parties in which video games were the main focus. "I am the best of the best, Mom. I won't even play with everyone. If they can't beat the second-best guy first, I don't bother. They have to beat him first." This was all silly college antics, but I was happy to hear that school was more than drudgery, and that Mike was enjoying his life.

Christmas break was approaching, and Mike began to come home on weekends occasionally. The three of us watched the morning news as we drank our wake-up coffee. One morning, the subject was terrorism and soft targets such as schools. Mike looked at me confidently and said, "Mother, I want you to know that if something really bad should occur, and we happened to lose communication, I don't want you to worry about me. I'm a very smart person and I'll find my way back to you." Those words remained in my memory, echoing in my mind, and later became my greatest hope. The terrorists to come would not be from the Middle East.

"Mom, let's go someplace warm for Christmas break. I won't always be with you." Another haunting remark. But at the time, it all made sense to me. Mike would go on with his life and one day leave us, to go on his own adventures. We decided on Miami, but Mark was worn out from teaching the first semester and didn't want to drive the 24 hours it would take to get to Miami.

"You two go. Enjoy yourselves. I'm going to get some rest!"

The day after Christmas, we got in the car for the long journey to Miami. We stopped in Atlanta, the halfway point, for a good night's sleep and continued the second leg the following day. I preferred to drive because I am a virtual "control-freak" in the car. Our seven-day visit with my nephew unfortunately did not provide the sunshine we expected, but daily, we enjoyed many adventures. We shopped, ate at shoreline restaurants, took a trip to the Keys, visited the ocean, and Mike went deep-sea fishing to fulfill his own dream. Even cloudy skies with seventy-five degree weather was better than northern Ohio's winters! The trip back was much the same, with a stop in Atlanta for sleep. The only difference was, on the way home, I asked Mike if he could drive for the last two hours.

"I'm running out of steam, Mike."

"Sure, Mom, I'll be happy to drive."

Nothing had seemed unusual throughout the entire vacation except one thing: Mike had his head-phones on, listening to music, for almost the entire trip. I had thought, *He must have a lot on his mind about his future.*

We encountered torrential rain, on the second day, hammering and pounding for most of the way home. We were lucky that the weather was unusually warm; otherwise, it could have been sleet. As we approached Lima, Ohio, for the last fill-up of gas and coffee, I asked Mike if he could take over now. Mike willingly took over the wheel, but my reprieve only lasted fifteen minutes.

"Mom, I don't know what's going on, but I feel over-caffeinated. I don't feel comfortable driving your van in this rain. Are you mad, Ma?"

"No, Mike, pull over. I can do it." Later, I could see the tremors that were developing in his hands. It wasn't caffeine, but that was what he would blame them on. The disease started right before my eyes, in January of 2005. I couldn't recognize the facts because the truth was veiled.

"Mike, maybe you should consider switching to decaffeinated coffee and colas," was my mothering response.

Second college semester didn't begin until the second week of January. Mike began to come home sometimes, mid-week and almost always on the weekends. While it was a joy and a pleasure to have him show up unexpectedly, I wondered what might be wrong.

"Mike, are you getting along with your friends?"

"Mom, they don't seem to care about anything important."

Mike's room-mates were busy making plans for the next school year, drawing straws for the rooms that would be available in their new apartment. Unfortunately, Mike had drawn the shortest straw, and got the worst room available. He told me that he had been accommodating in the past, and felt that this was an unfair assignment. Nonetheless, he asked us to sign a 12-month lease, with a huge down-payment required on the spot. We wrote the check and signed the lease agreement. Looking back, I realize that Mike was having mild delusions of grandeur. His ideas were hugely important and his internal goals remained unexposed to us. He was a great thinker and his friends had suddenly become shallow and uncaring about major and significant issues.

My cell phone continued to be our main source of communication. As the mother of an only child, I didn't want to intrude on his personal life, or wake him up from a sound sleep. My goal was to call on days that Mike had breaks, and should have been up and around. He was always sleeping until noon or later.

"Mike, were you partying too late?"

"No, Mom, I just can't seem to get enough sleep." I remembered how some of my siblings could sleep late, required more sleep than others, and didn't worry. Other times, later in the day, Mike was totally himself—alert, outrageously funny, and trying to make sense of the mad world of college. His anecdotes about his life and college adventures amused me. Always, he asked how Dad and I were doing. I then gave a report on our lives, knowing full well that his father called him just as often. I felt absolutely no sense of fear for his well-being.

May arrived and the second semester was over. Mike quickly moved his things home and planted them in the garage. They remained there without a plan to sort them or put them away in any sensible manner. They remained in almost exactly the same position for the entire summer. Mike appeared to be totally wasted. I thought that he was burned out on school because he'd had no break the previous summer. He slept late each day, showed no motivation to get a summer job, and drove his car incessantly, listening to his music. I was working long hours each day and Mark was on vacation for the summer, so I should have relied on his observations. Mark told me that Mike wasn't engaging with other people and didn't show an interest in anything. I approached Mike and questioned him.

"Mike, you could have treatable depression. You're sleeping all the time. Do you feel depressed?" Mike denied any feelings of depression. "Mike, are you taking drugs? You can tell me anything." This question was followed by loud and raucous laughter.

"Mom, I'm shooting up heroin!"

Of course I knew that he wasn't, but still insisted, "Mike, do you think that it might be a good idea to go see someone? You could have treatable depression with the pattern of your sleeping habits."

"Mom, I am not depressed, and I'm not taking drugs. I want to be an actor, and go to L.A."

My immediate response was No! I knew innately that he was a "babe in the woods" and that nothing good would come of this venture. *They'll eat you alive out there, Mike. You have no idea what you could be getting in to.* Mark and I had both hoped that since Mike was so close to finishing his degree, he would continue. Mark suggested that Mike use his business classes as a minor and look into theatre at the university. We became convinced that this was somehow 21-year-old angst and we could help Mike through it.

Mike clearly needed help in locating acting schools and agencies, and so I took on the banner. The first agency that we investigated was in a very shabby location in a big city. They had the largest advertisement in the phone book, and I thought this might be the best place to start. Mike pulled what I thought to be at the time, a childish shenanigan. He insisted on meeting with the agent by himself, dressed in James Dean style clothing – a white T-shirt and classic blue jeans. I know why he did this. He had been told for years that he looked like James Dean.

There was a long line of people showing up for the open-audition, but Mike's good looks got him an immediate invitation to have pictures taken by the photographer on staff. His photos were apparently not good and he was told that he looked "scared shitless" in front of the camera. Instead of giving up, Mike called the agent back and apologized for his weak imitation of James Dean.

Her reply was chastising, "That's twisted."

It was to my utter amazement when Mike asked me on two or three occasions if this agency had called me. "Why, would they call me, Mike?"

"Mom, they all looked Italian. I think that they could be associated with the mob."

"Mike, you are beginning to scare me. What you are saying sounds delusional. Those people forgot about you the minute you couldn't perform for the camera. They couldn't care less about you. Michael, you're not hearing voices, are you?"

"No, Mom, I am not hearing voices."

And, he wasn't.

I thought that immaturity and vanity had caused this foible. I explained to Mike that this was truly a silly act, but that I didn't like the looks of the building or location, right from the beginning. "We'll research other agencies, Mike. We need to find one that at least looks reputable. Next time, be yourself!"

We did find a reputable talent agency that offered modeling and acting lessons in a large city about two hours away from our home. This agency boasted that they had good connections with big agents on both the east and west coasts. Plans were made for Mike to take modeling and acting lessons consecutively and then compete with hundreds of other young hopefuls from around the country, in a safe and structured environment. This sounded much more sensible than quitting college and taking off on a wild goose chase. Mike finally seemed at peace with our new-found plan and agreed to finish his degree. Mark and I were hopeful that we had found a solution to Mike's yearning and agreed to pay for his lessons, provided he stayed in college. For a while, everyone seemed happy and satisfied with the new road map.

The truth was, Mike was disengaging and changing. He began to drink copious amount of coffee and smoke cigarettes heavily. The smoking had us completely baffled as we remembered the years of struggling to keep his airways open. Each time that Mike had come home from college, I thought that he looked thinner.

"Mike, you're losing weight. Are you getting enough to eat?"

"Mom, I'm eating all the time. I think that my metabolism has changed from smoking."

"Cut down on that smoking, Michael. It's not good for you, especially since you already have asthma." The occasional tremors in his hands were explained away in just the same manner.

"Mother, I am drinking too much coffee, and I'm smoking and using my Albuterol inhaler more often." I knew that his rescue inhaler could cause shakiness and was certain that this side-effect was the main culprit. Over a six month period, Mike dropped twenty pounds from his slightly chubby frame and was delighted with his newly svelte physique. Even Mark was not disturbed by his weight loss.

"Susie, leave him alone. Everyone in my family has fought the weight thing for years. It's OK for him to be the first thin Dunham. But still, I am very disappointed that he is smoking, after all that we have been through."

Mike went to our family doctor for his annual physical and to get his asthma medications refilled. He returned home from his appointment and announced that Dr. Waters told him that he was fit as a fiddle.

"Mike, did you tell Dr. Waters about the occasional tremors in your hands?"

"No, Mom, I forgot." But still, my mind was put to rest. Certainly, if there was anything major wrong with Mike, Dr. Waters would have picked it up. He was a sharp, young doctor. Mike did not actively pursue a job that summer, in spite of the fact that his father encouraged him repeatedly to put some applications in at local businesses. We live in a resort area, and the papers are always teaming with summer job opportunities. At the time, we were financially stable and comfortable, but certainly not wealthy people. Michael's lack of motivation to find summer work fell under the scrutiny of many relatives, on both sides of our family. There were indeed a number of arguments between Mark and me that summer. I believed that because Mike had never in his life shown any open signs of defiance, this new resistance was passive-aggressive behavior. We were forcing him to finish his degree, when all he really wanted was to get into acting.

"Mark, I think that Mike is really and truly burned out from not getting a break from school last summer and maybe we are asking him to fulfill our own dreams."

"Susie, you're wrong. You're working all the time and you're not here to see the changes."

A few things mystified me. We still shared morning coffee and the news, before I left each morning to see my customers. Occasionally, Mike exhibited a smile that I had never seen before. His mouth was wider and his lips were closer to his teeth. Sometimes, as he described his burning and anxious desire to be an actor, his eyebrows knitted up high and close together. This was my only child and I had contemplated his face thousands of times, but had never seen these expressions before. Did I imagine that his gait had changed as he walked across the room to get a refill of coffee? Why was he lifting his legs up like that when he walked? And why wasn't he swinging his arms? Did I imagine that his voice was delivered in a sing-song or monotone fashion? He had always been so animated. And yet, he seemed totally cognizant of the world, family events, and cared about other people. His dry but kind sense of humor was just as it had always been. For some reason, now that his dreams to be an actor were going to be realized with lessons and confirmation, he seemed completely at peace. In my mind, he appeared almost smooth.

But why were his teeth so discolored?

"Mike, your teeth are brown! You just had them cleaned by the dental hygienist a month ago. You want an image-oriented profession and yet your hair looks greasy." He quickly took a shower, brushed his teeth, and bought whitening strips.

Mea culpa. The signals were all there, but they were also intermingled with many meaningful and thoughtful conversations. I witnessed a whole lot of very sane behavior that made any of these signals and symptoms pale in comparison. Many of our relatives visited that summer of 2005. We hosted a small family re-union for Mike's male cousins, and no one could see anything wrong with him.

My little brother Tommy suffered a heart attack while attending a sales meeting in Chicago, shortly after Mike's 21st birthday, which was on July 10th, 2005. Mike heard the desperate phone calls from his Aunt Vickie as he came home from one of his long drives.

"Mom, wake up. Call Aunt Vickie. Uncle Tom had a heart attack." Once we were able to map out the location of the hospital, Mike hopped in the car with me, in the middle of the night, to take the five hour journey to see Tom and tell him that we loved him. Mike was my quiet and strong companion on this trip and showed nothing but love, support, and concern. He held his uncle's hand with compassion and told him he'd be alright and that we all loved him.

Mike was only able to attend his modeling lessons for two weeks before his psychotic break from reality. But during this time, he had a look of loveliness. His eyes showed a joyful serenity that I had never seen before. In retrospect, I would describe this look as one of mirthful wisdom. There was merriment in what he knew to be true. Sadly, I thought that he was simply happy to be on the path he had chosen for himself.

In my mind, what happened to Mike was not unlike the many Fourth of July celebrations we'd experienced when he was little. For years, I had driven into Michigan to purchase fireworks and dump far too much money into one night's festivities. We always started out with "spinners" and little cars and tanks that drove themselves and made small sparks, pops, and bangs. The evening activities escalated with bottle rockets and larger projectiles. The end of the evening, which we shared with family and neighbors, was the Grand Finale. In the dark, we shot off all the "big boys" out and above Lake Erie. Everyone clapped and shouted out the appropriate "ooohs" and "ahhhs." At 10:00, the grown-ups, with beers in hand, judiciously handed out sparklers to the children. By 11:00, the event was over. The kids were sent happily to bed and everyone was glad that no one got hurt.

For six months, there were little snaps, pops, and sparks going off in Mike's brain. They were there, but subtle. The chemical imbalances escalated. Bottle rockets and small projectiles. Louder, but not too loud. The Grand Finale came on July 29th in the year 2005. Sadly, no one was at home to watch or help when things went wrong.

It would be a very long time before we could even see a spark of life in him.

Chapter 3 – *Pieta* for Michael

In Italian, the word *pieta* means compassion or deep pity. Michelangelo's famous statue immediately comes to the minds of Christians throughout the world. "Sorrowful Mother" is almost a synonym. Mary's hands are lifted up in contemplation to God. "Why?" she asks. "Look what they have done to my Son."

I noticed as a child that the statue of the mother of Jesus is disproportionately large compared to the adjoined statue of her dead Son. I have heard that this may have been on purpose. Perhaps the statue was to have been placed on a hill and was designed to fool the eye of the beholder. Maybe it was to instill in the viewer's mind that this sorrowful mother was looking only at her Child, and that was why the Body of Christ was purposely carved in a smaller scale.

I am a Catholic of faith, if not of perfect performance. My pregnancy with Michael was threatened with complications, and I called on Mary for intercession, attached with a promise.

"Please, whisper in His ear, just like you did at the wedding feast. Tell Him that I need just this one child. I promise, I'll take very good care of him."

I was gifted with a beautiful baby boy, who acted like an angel all his life. Nineteen days after his twenty-first birthday, Michael became psychotic and was convinced that he was Jesus Christ, as in "The Second Coming." At first, it was nothing less than a surrealistic experience for me. It was unbelievable that a person of such integrity and intelligence could suddenly become so confused and disoriented.

Mary and I share the experience of being sorrowful mothers. Her son was Christ. My son was suffering from a tragic brain disorder because of chemical imbalances and disturbed wiring in his brain, and thought that he could save the world. There are many other "sorrowful mothers" of my kind. The delusion among schizophrenics that one is Christ is not uncommon. One point one percent of the population worldwide suffers from schizophrenia, and so as many mothers worldwide grieve for their children. My message is to explain the huge suffering of the person who is afflicted with this horrible disease. Understand the word *pieta* which means compassion, not a statue. The statue was named after an emotion.

The entities that tortured and tormented my boy were not Roman soldiers, but they were just as real. My *pieta* can only be defined by explaining what it was like to watch Michael's suffering along with his heroic and tenacious will to survive.

Part II – The Wrath Of God

Chapter 4 — 7:00 AM, July 29, 2005

"Get up, Mike. We have to go now! Our flight leaves at 10:30 and we're supposed to check in at the airport two hours early." Mike had promised to drop us off and pick us up when we got back in order to avoid the long-term parking fee.

Mark was about to have his dream fulfilled. He was turning fifty in less than a month. All he wanted was to take me to Seattle and Vancouver Island. I was always so busy with my business that I had neglected paying attention to one of the most important persons in my life, my husband and best friend.

"Do you want a party for your birthday?" I had asked him.

"No, I want you to go away with me."

"I'll go anywhere in the world with you. Let's plan it. Where would you like to go?"

Mike rolled sleepily out of bed at the last minute and requested fresh coffee in one of our Styrofoam "to go" cups. He attempted to wake up in the back seat of our car, drowsing and staring. Mark drove, read the map and gave multiple instructions simultaneously. The last minute confusion was almost too much to bear.

"Let's not get killed on the way to the airport, Dad," was about all that Mike had to offer as the caffeine brought him back to life.

The last hour's conversation was somewhat argumentative. Mark thought that Mike shouldn't have guests in our house while we were gone.

"Come on, Mark," I said to my cautious husband, "Mike's been away at college for three years. We live on Lake Erie! If he wants to have some friends over to enjoy the boat and build a bonfire, he should!" To my son, who had just turned 21 only nineteen days earlier, I said, "Michael, if you invite friends to the house and they drink anything, command them to sleep over. Don't let anyone drink and drive!"

Something hadn't been exactly "right" with Mike since the first of the year. I couldn't put my finger on it. He had what I described at the time as "inertia". He was like a machine that couldn't go forward, but also couldn't go backward. Our concerns had been safety issues, lack of a real plan, and how on earth were we going to cover him under our health insurance if he was not attending college? Mike still had some serious asthma and allergy concerns which required monitoring and medication. Throw in that he was a sheltered and immature 21 year-old. What confusion it had all been! But now the problem was solved. Mike was back on track to finish his degree in business and follow his own dream at the same time. With all of this turbulence behind us now, I felt that Mark and I could take this brief vacation with peace of mind.

We arrived at the airport on time. Because I am a detail-oriented person, I told Mike where our wills were located. I clearly remember telling him that we were off on an adventure and that he shouldn't worry about us. "We'll be back in five days and we'll have a wonderful time, Mike. We're sorry that we can't take you along this time because of your lessons. Next time, we'll take you with us."

Mike unloaded our bags and looked so forlorn that I wanted to cry. "I'm worried that something bad will happen to you and Dad, Mom."

"Nothing bad is going to happen to us, Mike." I knew that his concerns had to do with terrorists on airplanes. As I kissed him on his mouth and neck three separate times, I noticed once again that he smelled like me. For some reason, this seemed like an unusually significant goodbye. Mark followed suit. Father and son still kissed and embraced without shame in public. My biggest concern at that moment was whether he could make the few tricky turns back to the main highway that leads directly to our home. But why did this goodbye feel so different? Something just wasn't right. I could feel it.

We entered the airport after my final cigarette, registered our luggage, and tried to kill some time. I called Mike on his cell phone to make sure that he had made the correct turns. "I'm already on Route 2, Mom, I'm fine."

How could I have known that I was saying goodbye to my only child on that day in such a permanent way? How could I have ever believed that after this critical day, he would never again be the same as I had always known him? How could I have conceived that in our absence, uninvited visitors, "strangers," would intrude our lakefront home? We had been safe there. We never even locked our doors! Nonetheless, the strangers came. They took my son as hostage and stole his mind.

The strangers first seduced our son with promises of grandeur, but eventually turned cruel. The phones, computer, and TV were manipulated, but these events were only what I learned later. I was unable to reach Mike from thousands of miles away because he would not answer the phone which was "controlled." In our absence, Michael was relentlessly subjected to both auditory and visual hallucinations that were so secretive that even Mike's grandparents and friends in the neighborhood didn't know. How such a thing could be was inconceivable. For the five days that we were gone, Mike ate almost nothing and drank very little. Time had become irrelevant.

As Mark and I ferried through the Puget Sound, on our own journey to go whale-watching, our son was falling deeper and deeper into a world we knew nothing about. Our adventure could not compare to his. We were all suddenly in uncharted waters and the journey back would be long, painful, and full of unexpected twists and turns.

Chapter 5 – Our Return Trip, August 2, 2005

Even though the events of those painful days seem to have happened yesterday, it has taken me three years to have the courage to write about Mike's psychotic break from reality.

Our trip to Seattle and Victoria felt magical, a long-awaited opportunity to relax, and we took advantage of every opportunity. On the day of our arrival in Seattle, we walked the steep streets, explored the waterfront, and ate Alaskan king crab legs at a charming seaside restaurant. After dinner, we signed up to take a large ferry to Victoria, British Columbia, on the following day. The view of Mount Rainier with its snow-covered peak was spectacular from our cruise on the Puget Sound. The ferry was huge and luxurious with food and drinks available, hosting an enclosed cabin or the option to sit on the open deck.

In Victoria, we walked the streets, embracing the gift, art, and book shops along with the friendly bistro-style restaurants, flowers abundant and hanging or potted everywhere. Our first day in Victoria was devoted to touring Butchardt Gardens. Acres and acres of land were dedicated to displaying every available flower in every imaginable color, in mass presentations. It was hard to believe that a place like this existed on earth and not in heaven! A two-hour trip on a tour bus left just enough time to make reservations to go whale-watching on our third day in the Pacific Northwest.

This was the highlight of my trip. The medium-sized boat took us into the ocean, out of the Puget Sound, and departed at 1:00 PM. Usually, orcas are readily swimming, but we were the "lucky boat" and managed to see two humpback whales.

Ironically, it was a mother and her nearly grown male calf. The rules were that the boat must maintain a certain distance from the whales, and, if it is their whim, they will swim close to you. How close they came! How majestic, huge, and graceful they were as they surged deeply, rising again, over and over toward our boat! Just as these inquisitive, intelligent mammals surfaced 20 feet from our boat, and appeared to be looking at us, my film ran out. I could see their eyes. They were just as curious as their "watchers." I remember so well on that night, as Mark fell into an exhausted and dreamy sleep, I could not get to that wonderful "Land of Nod." I was far too excited and stimulated by the day's events, and tried to relax by reading all of the brochures and magazines about the area that were available in the hotel lobby. I decided that it was a good time to kneel down in reverence and pray. I recall "talking to God" saying, "Lord, today I have seen your majesty." I was sincere and profoundly worshiping of the real glory of God's works and creation. How little I knew what would await me when I returned home in forty-eight hours. For a while, I falsely believed that because I had truly seen God's grandeur, I was also supposed to see His wrath. And then, much later, as my senses have returned, I understood that only good things come from God, that He is the Author of creation, love, and mercy. I have held fast to this belief and my Catholic upbringing saved me from complete despair in the days to come.

Mike did not answer his phone for days. He left only one message on the very first day. "Mom, if the people from the modeling agency call you, will you have them call me back? It's pretty important that I speak with them. OK, thanks."

"Why would they call me?" I thought. I didn't get it. This message was delivered in a sing-song voice that I didn't recognize. This wasn't Mike's usual animated voice. What was up? I had refrained from calling at night because of the time difference and didn't want to wake Mike up. When I couldn't reach him during the day hours, I imagined that he was simply having a good time and was busy with friends. I also thought that he might have enjoyed having the house to himself.

Our last day was spent taking the luxurious ferry back to Seattle, then driving our rental car to a hotel near the airport which provided a shuttle to help us catch our flight home. I called Mike on my cell phone, and, finally, he answered. Mike announced that he was not going back to college. I couldn't help myself at this moment and literally flipped out.

"Mike, we just paid for your tuition and signed a 12-month lease for your apartment. What can you possibly be thinking?" Mike calmly replied that if he could only get the email address for a well-known screen director, he was sure that he could get into acting. I knew at this very moment that we had a big problem. This was simply delusional thinking. Mike told me that he had been feeling sick and had been nauseated, and somehow I understood that whatever was going on in him was a physical illness. There was no emotionality attached.

Mike's grandparents lived next-door and would have called us if they had noticed anything amiss in their first-born grandchild. But they hadn't seen Mike since the first day of our leave. Except for waving to Mike as he drove by, they had not seen him after this and were allowing him the privacy that he deserved as a 21 year-old young man. The only clue that they might have missed was delivered in a question from their long-term bridge playing friend who knew Mike well. Mike had slipped discretely into their garage to get a Diet Coke and was seen by only one of their bridge partners, who had asked, "What's wrong with Mike's eyes?" But, Mike had avoided contact with his grandparents, so they couldn't possibly have understood the question. For all they knew, Mike's "allergy eyes" had been noticed, once again.

On this evening, I called Mike again, but received no answer. I thought, "There is a problem awaiting me. Did Mike get into some drugs? Has he been taking drugs? I am thousands of miles from home. What can I do from here? I'll take care of this when I get back."

On August 2ⁿᵈ 2005, we boarded the plane in Seattle that would take us to Chicago, where we had an hour's layover before our final return flight to Cleveland. At 8:15 PM, we stopped in a bar at O'Hare Airport to have a drink and kill some time before our next flight. Mark called Mike once again, this time to remind him to pick us up at Cleveland Hopkins Airport at 11:30 PM, but there was no answer. We boarded our second flight, hopeful that Mike was simply busy. The flight went as planned and by 11:30 PM, we sat at the curb with our travel bags, waiting for Mike to pick us up. He didn't show. Over and over and over, Mark called Mike and left messages to come to get us. Mike finally answered his phone. My hugely responsible boy told his father, "Sometimes you just have to take care of yourself, Dad."

"What the hell's the matter with you? Get off your ass, get in the car, and pick us up!" Mark retorted, as he paced back and forth anxiously.

Mike did get in his car, but kept getting lost. He tried to get to us three times, but because signs such as "Route 6" said to him, "come in here" or some other strange message, Mike kept getting lost and returned home to a safe place.

Finally, on Mike's fourth try to come to Cleveland airport, I took the phone from my sincerely aggravated husband. I knew enough that this was not the moment to panic.

"Something's wrong, Mark. Let me speak to Mike. Mike, where are you now? Tell me the name of the sign that you are currently seeing." Mike was able to read the sign and I figured out at least he was heading east. "What's the next sign? ...What's the next? ...What's the next?" He was still going in the right direction. I directed him to take a quick right on Route 57, then another quick right into the parking lot of a furniture store that I had called on for years. "Park your car in this parking lot, Mike.

We'll take a cab to meet you. Everything will be OK. Just stay there, where I told you to go, and rest."

"OK, Mom."

We had exactly eighty dollars left in both of our wallets. We hailed a cab and asked the cab-driver if he could take us to this place about twenty minutes away for eighty bucks. The driver appeared to be of Middle Eastern origin and spoke little English. I was sorry that we didn't have anything left for a tip. At 3:30 AM, we arrived at the appointed place and saw our car. Mike was standing quietly outside the car, with eyes that looked bewildered and overcast. We advised Mike to get into the back seat to rest, and Mark drove all of us home. Mark began to ask a hundred questions about this fiasco which Mike seemed incapable of answering.

"Just get us home," I said quietly. After unloading the bags into our house, I said to Mike, "Let's go into the garage. Have a cigarette with me. Mike, what's been going on with you?"

"Mom, something strange has happened to me. I'm pretty sure that I am Jesus." The huge alarm went off in me. With my limited education, I knew that this was an ominous sign. I decided to agree with him to see if he would elaborate.

"Did you see angels, Mike?"

"Mother, I saw and heard thousands of them."

"That's good, Mike, and I want to tell you that I am a person of huge faith. Either you have had a profound religious experience, or you are as mad as a hatter."

"Mom, even crazy people know the truth," Mike calmly replied.

"You look so tired, Mike. Please go to bed and I'll come upstairs soon." As Mike ascended the stairs, I immediately went to my computer and turned it on. I spent two hours on the internet researching bipolar disorder because I didn't believe that he could possibly have schizophrenia and verbally describe his experiences this well. I remembered from my nurse's training that people who suffered from bipolar disorder had grandiose ideas and did hallucinate.

Around 6:00 AM, I decided to catch a few hours of sleep in our Lazy-Boy recliner. I perched this chair immediately in front of Mike's bedroom in case he decided to leave his room. He was on his left side, apparently resting. From my chair, his eyes appeared to be open. I believe at this very moment he was catatonic and simply "listening."

I fell into an exhausted sleep until 10:00 AM. It was suddenly August 3rd. Mark remained completely angry about Mike's total lack of responsibility and demanded that Mike cut the grass and return our boat to the dry-dock area which we rented. Astonishingly, Mike was able to accomplish these tasks! I couldn't believe that he was coherent enough to obey. Mid-afternoon, Mike persisted with his delusions about being the "Second Coming of Christ." I brought out our Bible and tried to read the book of Revelations to him. First he was Jesus, then David, and then Daniel. Because of my education as a nurse, I understood that he was experiencing "rapid associations."

I was totally horrified by this psychotic behavior and left the house to make an urgent call to our family doctor's office. On my way out of the neighborhood, I ran into my mother-in-law who greeted me and asked about the trip.

"Nancy, our vacation was great. Right now, I am going to make an important phone call. I'll be back in twenty minutes. Would you then come over and have a look at your grandson?" She agreed and showed up in exactly twenty minutes.

I drove two miles away, and parked my car at a gas station to speak privately on my cell phone. I wanted to make an appointment with Dr. Waters immediately. Linda, our beloved office nurse adored Mike. She listened to my concerns, reported them to Dr. Waters, and quickly relayed our doctor's message. *Take Mike to the closest hospital emergency room. We can't handle his problem in this setting.*

My sixth sense had told me that Mike was paranoid and would not agree to the idea of hospitalization. Somehow, I had the sensibility to make my initial plea away from anyone who could overhear my conversation. Now, it became clear that I had to convince others in our family that Mike had a serious problem and that he needed immediate help. When I returned, Mike's grandmother was there. "Mike, tell Grandma who you are."

"Grandma, I am Jesus. I am God. I am the wrath of God." Mike stood up in an entirely perplexed manner and looked profoundly at the palms of his hands. I understood he was searching for his own stigmata, but found no bloody nail marks. It was suggested by Mark and his mother that it might be a good idea to take Mike to dinner and a movie to help him snap out of this. This naïveté would only cause treatment to be postponed.

My instincts as a nurse to gently guide family members to recognize Mike's symptoms and to get them to acknowledge the reality of the situation had failed. It was only then that my instincts as a salesman kicked in. I thought to myself, "You need to go directly to the buyer and decision-maker."

Finally, on the next evening, I talked directly to Mike. "Michael, it appears to me that you have not slept well in a long time. How about we go to the emergency room and get you a nice shot to help you get a good night's sleep?" This was all trickery for him, and for his father and grandmother, who simply didn't get it. Mike was really ill, but somehow bought this idea. He must have been exhausted because my "sales presentation" was short and to the point.

Mark signed Mike into the emergency room and filled out the necessary paperwork as I quietly gave the history of the past week and Mike's symptoms to the charge nurse. Mike's eyes retained that blank and empty look, and he seemed oblivious to anything except the promise of a "good- night's sleep." We were lucky to be greeted by Dr. Kelley, a nice Irish ER doctor. I was dressed in mismatched, although clean clothes, with no make-up, wearing my glasses instead of my contact lenses because of lack of sleep. Dr. Kelley was clearly astute about what the problem could be. First, he ordered a blood test to rule-out illegal drugs.

Dr. Kelley returned to our cubicle within an hour. After ordering an injection of Ativan, which is a sedative, he announced to us that Mike was "clean" of any drugs whatsoever.

"Oh my God," I said, "This is very bad news." I told him that I had been a nurse long ago. He took me away from Mark and Mike, brought out a box of tissues and let me cry. I explained the entire situation and apologized for my appearance. "I don't usually look this disheveled, doctor." He kindly said that he could tell that and was calling in a professional who would give us advice on the next step.

The social worker came within thirty minutes, interviewed Mike privately, and then advised us that Mike was having a psychotic episode and was "thought blocking." He told us that Mike needed to go to a psychiatric hospital and offered to send an ambulance for the transport. I don't know where this wisdom came from, but we demanded to drive Mike ourselves. We didn't want Mike to become frightened or to be restrained in any way, and wanted to keep this terrible situation low-keyed.

We left the local hospital and headed for the psychiatric hospital, forty minutes away. Both of us made small talk as we drove along.

"This is the bridge we drove over for your birth," Mark said. "We're taking you to a hospital where they can help you, Mike. Everything will be alright."

I remembered well that trip from long ago, huffing and puffing and panting as we anticipated bringing the first breath of life to our baby. I hoped that this new hospital could restore that life which had been so difficult to guide in. Mike was calm the entire trip. It wasn't until we parked that he balked.

"I want to run, Mom."

"Don't run, Mike. You have a chemical imbalance. These people will help you. We'll get this fixed and everything will be OK. Do what they say."

The rest of the evening was even more surrealistic. They were expecting us. After a brief phone call from the admitting desk that had announced our arrival, we marched in like the Three Musketeers, Mark and me on each side of Mike, and two armed guards following closely behind us. I couldn't believe what was happening! My gentle and noble son, who had never committed a crime, was being escorted by armed security guards. I wondered, "Why were the guns necessary? Mike hadn't shown any signs of violence or resistance." I also knew that men who carried guns were prepared to use them, and sometimes mistakes were made.

We stayed to help Mike as he willingly admitted himself for treatment. I knew enough to make sure that he signed the "Release of Information Form" so that we could have access to the results of his tests and progress. I understood that he was now 21 years old, and in spite of the fact that Mark's health insurance paid for his hospitalization, we had no rights to information without Mike's written consent.

On August 5th, 2005, at 5:00 in the morning, we went home to our empty nest. We had been sleep-deprived for days, confused and terrified. Our house was missing our one essential person who was our beautiful only child. In spite of the fact that Mike had never intentionally harmed a person or thing in his life, he had been treated as a potential criminal. That night, we slept from sheer exhaustion. Our brutal experience with "the system" would unfold quickly, just like one nasty peel after another of a rotting onion. This was the landmark date of the beginning of our nightmare as parents of a child with a mental illness. "If this could happen to Mike, it could happen to anyone," I thought, as I fell into oblivious sleep. That almost unconscious deliberation was the beginning of my wisdom on mental illness.

Chapter 6 – The Next Morning

"Mark, will you please make me some coffee?" For over 23 years, this had always been my clue that I was awake and ready to talk. It was 10:00 AM and we had only slept for four hours, but neither of us could sleep any longer. The first thought that came to my mind as I awoke was, "This is not just a bad dream. This is real. It really happened. Mike has schizophrenia. I simply can't believe it."

I rushed into the bathroom to vomit. I vomited into the sink because I couldn't make it to the toilet. This visceral reaction to my "first thought of the day" continued for many, many, next mornings. It was as involuntary as a hiccup, but far more predictable. I had seen the devastation of this disease along with the long-term disastrous side-effects of medications. Reality always set in after that, even before the first cup of coffee, and this was simply "the first next morning."

In our usual ceremonious way, Mark handed me my favorite cup, filled with fresh coffee. He sat across from me in our living room and for a long time, we said nothing. We were like cows taken to the slaughter-house that were first clubbed on the head and dazed, before the sharp knife came to cut our throats. We simply looked at each other. Finally, Mark put his hands to his face and openly cried.

"I can't believe that this happened to Mike."

"I can't either."

We cried together, but in our own separate locations. He sat on his recliner and I on the sofa. There was no hugging or kissing that could comfort either one of us. This was simply a long session of sharing our individual grief with a steady stream of quiet tears.

"What are we going to do?" I asked.

Finally, Mark looked me directly in the eyes and said, "You tricked Mike. You knew that if we took him to a hospital, they would want to admit him."

"Mark, Mike is really terribly sick. We can't handle this kind of illness. He needs to be in a safe place where they can monitor his medication. We can't do that here." I knew that Mark simply wanted his son right next to him. I understood his anguish.

In the midst of our mutual grief, "the light suddenly went on." So "this" was what all of Mike's confusing behavior had been leading up to. Why didn't we know more about this disease in advance? Why didn't we know what to look for? Could we have prevented this with medication? How could we have failed Mike so miserably? We thought that we were intelligent people. How could we have been so absolutely ignorant and stupid?

Always, in the middle of a tragedy, practicality must set in. Mark had taken a summer job coaching tennis for his high school and was expected to be at the tennis courts by noon. We were informed the previous night about visiting hours, which were quite limited. We could only see Mike from 12:00 to 1:30 and from 6:00 to 7:30. We both cleaned up as best as we could. Mark went to coach his team and I went to visit Mike. Mark and I would visit Mike together later in the day. Mark had no other choice.

We both limped through that first day of Mike's hospitalization. The horror of the disease, the horror of the system, if one could call it a "system," and the horror and dread of the future were ominous in both our minds.

I drove to the hospital alone, my mind racing. I didn't believe that any good outcome was possible for this disease. I knew it was schizophrenia, even though the final verdict had not yet been given. How was I going to take care of Mike now, when I had to work? How was I going to provide for Mike after my death? How was I going to tell my family? I knew that it would hurt them because I understood their strong love for me, and I for them. My seven siblings and I are all "connected at the hip." We had all been through the deaths of our parents, major illnesses, and other tragedies as a unit, a team, a club. Ours was an exclusive club that offered no open memberships. Only the eight of us could belong.

As I parked my car in the hospital parking lot, the very obvious thoughts came to mind: *how could it be that two parents tried this hard, made this many sacrifices, and have it all turn out like this?* We thought that we were almost at the "finish-line" on the racetrack. Just one more year of college and acting lessons would launch our kid into a world that held endless opportunities. We thought that we would have a number of grandchildren, whom we could bounce on our knees, sing to, read to, and surprise with presents. I saw all of our dreams slipping away. What a "bad trick" this disease was. Just as we were getting older and tired and thought that our job was almost done, everything that we had strived for and worked for had been apparently robbed from us. All of my conceived realities came crashing in at once. I pulled myself together. First and foremost, I wanted to see Mike. I wanted to believe that he really was in a safe place and that they were treating him well.

It was the hottest day of August with the highest humidity that I can remember. I walked into the hospital and approached the front desk to ask directions to the psychiatric unit. I was breathless from the heat, and couldn't quite remember from the previous night exactly how to get to Mike's room. I was dressed in clothes that would be appropriate to call on my furniture dealers and had decided that it was important to project a professional image. I didn't want the attending nurses to think that I was a mother who was uncaring or had no clue as to what was happening.

Chapter 7 – Inside the Double-Locked Doors

As I approached the double-locked doors, which required a doorbell announcement and phone system to be admitted, I was in for a huge education about a psychiatric unit. I was so disappointed! But, I was equally glad that I had divorced myself from nursing before I had become so disenchanted and burned out. After Mike's first hospitalization in a psychiatric unit, I was truly sad for the whole profession of nursing.

I was buzzed inside the double-locked doors by a very large man whom, initially, I thought was a male nurse. He was totally unwelcoming, quiet, distant, and staring around the unit. I asked what room Mike was in. I'd been told to bring in some comfortable leisure clothes the evening before. I entered Mike's room and placed his clothes in the bedside stand. I found him lying quietly on his side, and his eyes displayed a condition called "nystagmus," which means rapid lateral eye movements. Other than the rapid lateral eye movements, he didn't move a muscle and was apparently catatonic. Immediately, a female nurse came in and told me that I was not allowed to be in Mike's room. I wondered how she expected me to deliver his clothes.

"Mike," I called, "can you come out to the lounge? They won't let me visit with you in your room." Mike dutifully got up and came out to the lounge, but only wanted to lie down. I stayed for only fifteen minutes on this first visit because Mike seemed clearly exhausted. The lounge had very uncomfortable, institutional furniture, and I wondered why it had been purchased because it seemed purposefully uninviting. There certainly was nothing appealing about this prison-like environment. I attempted to ask Mike simple questions. "Did you have a good breakfast?" It seemed to take at least two or three minutes for him to answer, after I repeated the question.

"I don't know. I can't remember."

I continued with similar, simple questions, which only resulted in the same confused and very delayed responses. Finally, Mike responded in his usual polite manner, which remained totally intact.

"Mom, can I please just go back and lie on my bed?"

"Sure, Mike, get some rest. Dad and I will be here this evening."

Defiantly, I entered Mike's Isolation Unit to tuck him in bed. He had a private room with a camera mounted to the wall to view his every movement, or in his case, "non-movement." The bathroom mirror was made of a shiny stainless steel plate so that it couldn't be broken and provide sharp glass shards. Belts and shoelaces were also prohibited, as well as any other item that held the potential for self-harm. I covered Mike up with a flimsy bed blanket that provided no real warmth, and thought that the temperature was so frigid that I should have been able to see my own breath. I had been told that Mike was in a "suicide prevention room," by the charge nurse.

I was in total shock and disbelief. I watched Mike as he crawled into his bed and lay, once again, on his side. He was a 21-year-old man, but he looked so frail. I now observed how skinny his legs had become. Why hadn't we been able to put all of these "clues" together? Were we simply stupid people? He looked like a baby bird that had unfortunately fallen from the nest before it was capable of flying on its own, simply waiting to die – just breathing, just staring, just waiting for the inevitable to come.

As I left, I approached the desk of the nurse's station to ask about Mike's condition. "What's been done?" Mike had already been through a gamut of tests early that morning, including blood tests and an MRI. All had proven to be normal. I asked what medications Mike was receiving, and the nurse reported that Mike was receiving Resperidol, an antipsychotic, along with Lithium, which is used to manage bipolar disorder. This female nurse was factual, remote, and distant. There didn't appear to be one ounce of kindness within her to identify with my shock, horror, and pain. Briefly, she asked what had happened. I volunteered that Mike thought he was Christ and that he had seen and heard angels.

"You should be grateful that they weren't devils," she curtly replied.

How little did I know at this time that "the devils" would later come to visit and torture my poor boy!

As I was "buzzed out" of this unit, by the same large man who had buzzed me in, it seemed as if he was staring at me. Was I feeling paranoid? I had never been a paranoid person. It had always been to my own detriment that I was never able to tell when people didn't like me. I had been raised by my loving family with complete acceptance, and it had never been easy for me to identify any other motives in people. I passed the "male nurse" with a lowered head, and wondered, *Does he think that I'm responsible for this train-wreck?*

I was too confused and overwhelmed at the time to guess the truth. This "male nurse" wasn't a nurse at all. He was only an orderly who had been hired purely because of his size and ability to pose as an ominous threat to anyone who "stepped out of line." He was simply the "bouncer" in this cold tavern that served nothing other than chemical cocktails, and had no interest in exchanging friendly banter with their patrons.

As I drove home, the trembling began. This was no longer shock, horror, and denial, but real fear. Practicality set in, once again. Mike was in a psychiatric unit and unable to communicate with me. I had not been back to work. There was still a mountain of laundry from our vacation and Mark still had to coach tennis. Everyone around me appeared to be in denial about how serious this was, or else they just didn't "get it." My faxes and emails were overflowing from our vacation, but I was overwhelmed by my need to attend to the current dilemma and crisis. I needed to talk to a good "steady head." I called my brother Jim.

Chapter 8 – First Call for Help

I called Jim on his cell phone, and luckily he answered. I often called all of my brothers regarding the furniture business and family matters. It was simply a miracle that he was in his car and answered his phone at this critical time.

"Jimmy, are you currently in a situation in which you can talk to me? I have something going on that is so large I can barely describe it. If there was ever a time in my life that I needed you most, this is it. It's huge and terrible, Jim," I sobbed.

"What's going on Suz?" Rapidly, I spilled my guts.

"Susie, I know that you don't want to believe this about your Mike, but I think your boy got into some drugs."

"No, Jimmy, it's already been disproven. Please keep this information in confidence. Don't tell our brothers and sisters what's happened to Mike. I'll tell them when the time is right." I was particularly concerned about our youngest brother, Tommy, who had recently suffered a heart attack and had three stents implanted under dire circumstances. "Please Jim, keep this our secret." He promised that he would, and I knew that I could trust him.

Jim drove four hours the very next day to visit Mike in the psychiatric unit of the hospital. He couldn't believe what he was seeing. He maintained his composure and quietly told me, "All business matters will be taken care of through me." Somehow, my phones, faxes, and emails shut down quickly and mysteriously. Jim alerted our superiors at the factory that I had an extraordinary circumstance and tragedy going on, and had all calls and service issues directed to him. I couldn't believe the silence that followed. It was almost eerie.

Jim took care of me during the early traumatic and mournful period. He later told me that for the next two years, he cried upon waking up every morning. It was purely and simply so unbelievable. He had seen first-hand that a beautiful and bright young man's brains had been scrambled.

Chapter 9 – Three Days in the Hospital

I drove to the hospital alone each day for an early visit. Mark and I drove together each evening, and Mike's grandparents came each evening as well. Mike appeared to "come alive" a little, later in the day as each day passed.

"Mom, when can I come home?" While he still seemed vague and withdrawn, Mike didn't appreciate his confinement. He often asked, "When will you get me out of this place? They won't let me outside. I can't even have a cigarette. I want to be at home, Mom."

After the first 24 hours, Mike had been released from the "Isolation Room" and given a room within the general population of the ward. Apparently, he was determined to be of no danger to himself or others. While I observed the behaviors of the other patients and understood that they had very serious problems and illnesses, I thought, "In many ways, they seem more human than their caregivers." The nursing staff seemed distant, remote, and unfeeling. The sickest of patients attempted to converse with Mike and me as well. They all knew why they were there. We were simply new to this whole idea. I was extremely humbled by their honesty. On the second morning, I learned from Dr. Kim that Mike had been taken off Lithium. When I asked why, he told me that he determined that Mike didn't need it. I knew right away that we were no longer dealing with bipolar disorder. It was schizophrenia.

Mike's tests showed that he did not have a brain tumor, thyroid problem, or any evidence of illegal drugs in his system. This information was given to me by the head nurse. Michael was on only one medication now, Resperidol, for his acute psychotic episode.

"How long will it take for this drug to kick in?'

"It'll take time."

I rephrased my question, "How long does it usually take?"

"It varies," she responded.

Once more, I asked, "In your professional experience, what is the average period of time that it takes to see results?" She put her head down and continued to write whatever she was writing before I had approached the desk. I stood there for some time, waiting for an answer. She never again raised her head to address me. I knew that I had been dismissed.

She didn't know that I had previously worked as a nurse. I searched my memories and hoped that I had never treated any family member with such little regard. I thought, *My Lord, if you have any other disease, you are offered information, treatment options, and possible outcomes. If you are undergoing surgery, you are alerted to every possible complication that might occur from either the surgery or the anesthetic. You are required to sign off on a consent form before anyone will consider treating you.*

The more I thought about it, the more horrified I became. This same nurse told me a story about a woman, a professional person who had suffered a stressful event in her life. "She came into our ward, wearing a salad bowl on her head, and sat here, saying nothing for two weeks. Later she came out of it. This could just be a bump in the road for your son."

I felt indignant. I thought, *You actually believe that stressful events caused this disease? You stupid shit! Mike had a perfect life! This is clearly a neurological illness.* I now understood the tremors in his hands. I wondered how she could explain away neurological symptoms. Was she advocating some article she had read in a nursing publication or a women's magazine? Either way, I thought that she didn't have a clue and certainly didn't belong in her position.

Then I realized that even the most educated of nurses, who worked on these wards, didn't always know what they were talking about, and had preconceived ideas about "what might upset a person's chemistry." What a disappointment this was! Where were they getting their information? Was this the way it was with everyone?

I was able to connect with Dr. Kim at least once a day during my visits. "I want to take Mike home, Dr. Kim. It appears to me that all that is happening here is that the nurses are giving medicine. Mark and I can take care of Mike at home and administer the same drugs."

Dr. Kim relented on the third day and then followed with directives. "You will need to follow up with a psychiatrist. I can take care of Mike in my office, or you can choose the psychiatrist of your choice."

"I don't know any psychiatrists, Dr. Kim. Why wouldn't we trust you to take care of our son? You have taken care of him so far."

The next morning, Mike was released to our care. He looked mostly like himself and was making sense in what he said, but I noticed that his eyes looked too bright.

"Mom, take me home. I never want to go back to this fucking place again." I agreed but was quite surprised by his unusual language. Mike didn't favor cursing or swearing, in spite of the fact that I routinely swore like a sailor.

I listened as my 21-year-old was given verbal instructions and signed his discharge forms. The instructions were simple:

1)   Take medicine as prescribed.
2)   Do not take any vitamins or herbal supplements.
3)   Do not drink alcohol.
4)   Follow up with Dr. Kim in 5 days.

I was invisible as far as the head nurse was concerned. No educational packet was given to us, and no support system such as NAMI (National Alliance on Mental Illness) was acknowledged. She did casually mention on discharge that there was a wealth of information on the internet about mental illnesses. First I wondered, *What is she afraid of? False promises?* Later, I realized that for the poor and uneducated, who did not have access to a computer, there were absolutely no "discharge resources." What happened to these people?

I was really glad to get my kid out of this cold, unfeeling, and apparently unhelpful environment. As we drove home, I was happy to have my son in the passenger seat, right next to my side. I believed that with medication, we could squash this unhappy event quickly. But that was not to be. The nightmare continued.

Chapter 10 – Two Days and One Night at Home

We drove over the bridge that crosses the bay that leads directly to our home on the lake.

"Mike, are you hungry?"

"Yes Mom, I am."

"What would you like to eat?" Mike wanted a meatball sandwich, so we stopped at a fast food restaurant. Mike took only one bite and then folded the sandwich back into its wrapper.

"Mike, was there something wrong with your sandwich?"

"No, I guess I'm just not that hungry." Later I would learn that the voices were commanding him to eat only melon.

"It's a beautiful sunny day, Mike. Don't you think so?" Mike stared straight ahead, now with intense eyes.

"I want to drive my car, Mom. I want to listen to my music."

"Mike, for right now, you can't drive, but I'll be happy to drive you around, and you can play anything that you want on the radio."

We went for three or four drives in the car on that first day, listening to Mike's contemporary music. Some of it I liked, but the volume was a problem for me. Was he trying to drown out something? Mike continued to deny hearing voices.

I remembered earlier in the year how Mark had questioned Mike about the seven hundred dollars on his credit card, most of which came from gas stations: "How can you be using this much gas?"

"Are you buying beer and cigarettes for your friends?" I had asked.

"No, Mom, I just like to drive my car and listen to my music." Since Mike had come home from college in the spring, this compulsive driving continued, resulting in many long trips in the middle of the night while my husband and I were sleeping. Mark had tried over and over to tell me that Mike was disengaging, but I had refused to believe it. I had insisted that Mike was being forced to finish his degree, while all he really wanted to do was study acting. In my mind, Mike was pretty much a perfect kid, and nothing could have convinced me otherwise.

On this day, in between these drives, Mike lay on his bed quietly as I continued the laundry, dishes, and preparation of supper. But his agitation increased as the day wore on. Mark had come home from his coaching position and tried to communicate and make sense with Mike. This was strictly a lost cause. With little or no sleep for days, Mark and I were desperate to close our eyes, just for a few hours. By bedtime, Mike was fully agitated and pacing. I didn't believe that he was totally aware of his surroundings, and hid the keys to his car behind a vase on the china cabinet. Not only was he fully aware of everything that was going on in his head, but also completely aware of what was going on in the household. He knew exactly where I had placed his car keys and was waiting for an opportunity to grab them.

In spite of the fact that Mike was twenty-one years old, we invited him to sleep between us, holding his hands to comfort and reassure him that everything would be OK. Mike had taken his Resperidol at 8:00 PM and promptly thrown it up. Later, we would learn from Mike that the "voices" told him to gag himself to get rid of the drug.

Every fifteen minutes, Mike got up for a cigarette. I followed him and had one with him, then kindly tried to urge him back to bed. After two hours, there was no point in trying. He was fully awake with eyes blazing. He had become defiant now. He lit a cigarette and sat in Mark's recliner, tapping the ashes on the floor. I gently coaxed him to use a plate for the ashes and was met with rebellion. When Mark came out of our bedroom to intervene, Mike stood up and drew out his lighter to set afire Mark's tennis coaching schedule. Mark asked, as he stomped out the fire, "Mike, why are you doing this? You could set the house on fire."

"It's just a thing, Dad." I wondered if this wasn't a profound thought and if it was uttered because Mike was comparing it with the loss of his mind.

"Mike, we have to live somewhere," Mark replied. Mark thought that he had settled things down and returned to our king-sized bed. I watched.

Mike proceeded out the door to our second-story deck and grabbed the large blue plastic bucket that had served to ice up beverages for his male-cousin family reunion, only six weeks earlier. He turned it over and stood on it, raising his arms up to the sky. I was absolutely certain that he was about to dive off the deck to his death.

"I won't let you jump, Mike!" I leaped toward him, grabbed his T-shirt from behind and pulled on him with all my weight. I was able to bring him down, directly on top of me.

"Is that what you thought I was doing?" my gentle boy asked, with a sarcastic smile that I had never seen before. Later I learned that he had "stopped all wars and healed the entire world from cancer."

I know that psychosis is an absolute detachment from reality, but I believe that there are indeed levels of psychosis. Around three o'clock in the morning, Mike's eyes changed again. They were suddenly the eyes of a dead man walking in this world, not really seeing or comprehending. In this new dream-state, with his hands in front of him like a sleep-walker, he paced the house, touching walls, apparently unaware of my presence. I felt like I was in a Stephen King movie, and that someone had taken my son and exchanged him for this person who only remotely resembled him. This wasn't Mike! This was a changeling!

"Mark, get up! Get out here! Look at his eyes! Look at him! He doesn't even look like himself!" At this point, I was shrieking from the shock of it and crying. It occurred to me later that Mike couldn't distinguish between his own body and his physical surroundings.

Once again, Mark got up from his brief sleep and commanded Mike to go to bed. Mike's eyes changed back again. Mark never saw the "dead man's eyes." Now they were blazing and angry as Mike leapt past both of us to retrieve the keys to his car, which I had believed were well-hidden.

"Stop him, Mark. He might hurt himself!" Mark raced down the stairs and placed his hands on Mike's elbows to try to halt his running, but was thrown back by his son who was now a featherweight. I raced past Mark. Mike's car had been purposely parked in the garage with my car parked directly behind, on the driveway with the doors locked.

"Give me those keys, Mike! You're not going anywhere." He sat confidently in the driver's seat as I wrestled with him for the keys, pulling them from his hand. And then he was gone. He ran from me out the front door, and disappeared. Mark got into his car at 5:00 in the morning, searching the neighborhood and nearby roads. Just before sunrise, Mike showed up and stood on the dock with his arms raised to the heavens in a "V," commanding the universe from our lakefront home. Eventually, we were able to lure Mike inside before the neighbors awoke.

"Please, Mike, go to bed, and try to get some rest," we begged.

Mark stood guard and allowed me to sleep for a few hours; but the next day was more of the same. I drove Mike several times in the car, listening to current hits on the radio. Mike stared straight forward, again with intense eyes, and refused to converse. The afternoon came and Mike's grandmother came over to visit once again. The TV was tuned to CNN, and Barbara Starr was the reporter.

"See, she knows what's going on," Mike said, as he pointed to the television. Later he returned to his room and alternately turned to his own computer or TV, looking deeply into the screens of each and touching them as the communication continued.

By the time that Mark returned from his coaching practice, I was frantic. No one understood the magnitude of this desperate situation.

"Mark," I said, "Mike has to go back to the hospital. This medicine isn't working. He needs help. We can't give him the help that he needs here. He could hurt himself." Silently, I thought, *...and maybe us.* I didn't know at this time that Mark had secretly hidden all of the sharp knives in our kitchen, but this was the substance of my grief. How could it be that my fine young man who held my arm going up and down steps, opened doors, and pulled out my chair in a restaurant had the potential to hurt me? I began to cry as this awful thought occurred to me.

"I hate that psychiatric ward and so did Mike. You saw what happened! They drug people up and ignore them. They don't even speak to us. We can take care of our son here." Mark was absolutely opposed to taking Mike back to the hospital and defended his position very well. Mike never liked to hear us argue about anything. He came out of his room and, for a short period, appeared to be somewhat lucid.

"What are you fighting about?"

"Mom thinks that you should go back to the hospital, Mike. She thinks that you need more help," Mark replied.

"Mom, is that true?"

"Mike, I think that you are depressed and that they can help you." *I knew that wasn't the problem.* "Things aren't quite right, don't you agree?"

To my utter amazement, Mike agreed that he should go back to the hospital. We had been told at the last minute, by the discharging nurse, that we could bring Mike back if things weren't going well. We packed Mike's personal items and drove over the bridge, once again, to the hospital. We first went to the hospital emergency room, which took hours for a readmission to the psychiatric unit. We were then directed, with much less drama this time, no armed guards, to the unit.

This time, we knew where to go. Once again, Mike voluntarily committed himself. The admitting nurse was very dismissive of me and proceeded to ask only Mike questions which, in some cases, he was unable to answer. The hospital records were there from his last admission, and at least we felt confident that something valid was in place. Whether the admitting nurse asked him or not about signing a Release of Information Form for his parents is still unclear. I seriously doubt that she bothered to offer it or to explain it to Mike. In any case, that form was not signed.

We drove home in silence, fragmented people. We were faced not only with an illness, but a death and a war of sorts. There are all kinds of tragedies that parents must endure, but the loss of a child's mind seemed to be right there at the top.

Chapter 11 – Ten Days in the Hospital

It began like a rerun of a very bad program shown on television with more of the same behaviors from hospital personnel. The nurses remained guarded and sat behind the desk, dispensing pills and taking notes. Once again, Mike was placed in the "Isolation Room" with cameras posted over his bed and also in the bathroom. The same "male nurse" stood guard outside the nurse's station, constantly vigilant, watching every movement of both patients and family members with menacing eyes. It was more than unfeeling and unemotional – it was creepy.

The visits from our family remained the same. Since my phones, faxes, and emails from my customers had become silent, I was able to pay attention only to the matters at hand. I visited Mike, both afternoons and evenings, without distraction. Mark and his parents, again, came every evening. The token gift that Mark and I brought each time was food, because there was no other act of caring that we could think of at the time. We delivered restaurant food of Mike's choice each evening. Often, whatever he didn't eat was stolen by the other patients, but we didn't care. We considered it a donation to the patients who obviously had no visitors.

On my early visit of the very first day, Mike had returned to his catatonia, lying quietly on his bed, asking for nothing. Again, this was a re-run of a very bad TV program. Mike had little to say, was slow to respond to questions, and simply wanted to lie on his side and stare. This first visit was brief.

Mark and I returned for the evening visit together. Mark had dropped me off at the main entrance and parked the car. I proceeded to ring the bell to be admitted inside the double-locked doors. From there I was admitted to the isolation area through another set of locked doors. I announced myself to the nurse in charge and asked how Mike was doing that evening. She looked like a doe in the headlights and told me that she couldn't give me any information because I wasn't listed on the "Release of Information" Form. I replied that Mike had only recently been discharged and questioned why this form had not been signed by Mike. She held steadfast, no matter my apparent aggravation.

"This is strictly bullshit. I'll get that problem fixed right now," I said. I approached the familiar room and demanded, "Michael, come out here right now and sign this form!" Mike had the sense to ask what it was for, and I replied, "Without your written permission, Dad and I can't find out anything about you, your medications, tests, or your progress." Mike immediately signed the form with a hand that displayed major tremors. I was absolutely dumbfounded that the admitting nurse from the previous night had not emphasized the importance of the form. Had she even offered it and explained it, or did she simply gloss over this important document? Was she an advocate of anyone, whether a patient or family member? I didn't have a very long time to analyze these questions that were dominant in my mind. Quickly, I thought, *This is why I left nursing. None of you can think outside the box. You are all so ingrained in rules and regulations that you can't see past them and simply help people!* As for this current nurse, who was in charge, I wondered why she didn't simply offer to present the form to Mike and ask him if he wanted to sign it. She had to be coerced to do the right thing! What happened to parents who didn't possess a fighter's instinct? And what happened to their kids?

Mike immediately announced that he wanted to see a priest and that he needed an exorcism. I looked the charge nurse squarely in the eyes and asked, "Is there a priest on duty you can call?"

Staring at me with wide eyes, she dialed the phone. "He'll be here shortly," she timidly replied. This request must have fallen into the protocol of acceptable plans of action. I gazed deeply into her eyes, and, for the first time in this facility, announced that I had once been a nurse, which I had not mentioned up to now.

Mark arrived about ten minutes later, after parking our car a long distance away in the visitor's parking lot. I gave Mark a brief synopsis of what had transpired in the last ten minutes. We both entered Mike's isolation room, disobeying commands that we couldn't go in there, and held Mike's hands as we patiently waited for the priest.

"Mike, you have a chemical imbalance and what you are seeing and hearing and feeling isn't real. Medication will make this all go away," I said, with my knees knocking so hard that I thought I might faint and fall down.

Mike was trembling and crying, "Mom, Dad, there are devils inside me. They are making rushes go all the way from my forehead down my spine. They're making me eat my own brains. I can feel myself swallowing my own brains! I want to see a priest. I need an exorcism." The devils were "voices" that threatened to kill Mike if he even dared to divulge their presence. The kind angels who must have told him that he was God had become fallen angels. They tormented him, accused him falsely, threatened his life, and planned to stay a very long time.

Within ten minutes, a very kind-faced priest arrived at Mike's bedside. He introduced himself and asked Mike a few questions. He must have had some sort of education on these matters because as Mike explained his current dilemma with the devils, the good father quietly told Mike that this was all an illusion and that it wasn't real. Once again, I told Mike that he had a chemical imbalance in his brain and that medication would help him. The priest anointed Mike and together we prayed, touching Mike and later holding hands, asking God for relief from this terrible torment. Then the good father asked Mike if he wanted to go to confession and to receive Holy Communion. I looked at the priest with new horror and, for the first time in my life, spoke very forcefully to an ordained minister of the Catholic Church.

"Father, he is in no condition to make a good confession. Just give him Communion!" Somehow I had omitted the word 'please'. I believed that The Holy Eucharist would bring healing and that under these extraordinary circumstances, this Gift from God Himself was absolutely necessary. The priest did give Mike Holy Communion and Mike accepted God's Gift in a sideways, half-kneeling, reverent position. The priest offered me Communion and I replied that I had not been to confession or Mass in some time. Instead, he gave me a blessing and Mark as well, who is not a Catholic. That blessing was deeply needed and appreciated.

I would learn later that the helpful young priest came to visit Mike and to check on his progress at least two or three more times. I wondered how much he really knew about mental illness. Had he been as totally shaken as we were? Priests are usually very well educated, but how much time did the seminary devote to psychiatric disorders? In any case, he was there for us. He came promptly at the hour of our need and brought to Mike, on that first evening, a measure of peace. Mike calmed down, and we were able to go home for some rest after this gut-wrenching incident.

Mike was kept in the "suicide prevention room" for three days and then released to a double occupancy room within the general population of the unit. There he remained for seven more days. This time, we were not in such a hurry to bring him home. We wanted to see more improvement than from the last admission.

For the remainder of Mike's hospitalization, only two nurses stand out in my mind as truly caring individuals. The first was a fairly recently graduated registered nurse. She worked on the evening shift twice while Mike was hospitalized in the isolation area. I admitted that I had been a licensed practical nurse years before.

"What is it with the nursing staff here?" I asked her, "It's like they have no soul!"

"Susie," she said, calling me by my first name, "They have all been here too long. They're jaded. They believe that this ward is nothing but revolving doors for patients who get better, then go home, and quit taking their meds." She was young, pretty, friendly, and bubbling with enthusiasm.

"That won't happen with us," I replied. "If we can get Mike better, I never want to see this place again."

"The "second caring nurse" only worked once that I can remember, during the evening visiting hours. I was sitting on an uncomfortable sofa in the lounge, with Mike's head on my lap.

"Pull on my hair, Ma." This sounded absolutely awful to anyone who might have heard his request, but I knew what he meant. Mike had always loved a scalp massage. He liked to have his hair in big clumps, pulled gently away from his scalp, along with massage. So, I provided an old remedy for a good night's sleep. A kind nurse, who was probably almost exactly my age, noticed the steady stream of quiet tears run from my eyes, and left the barricade of the nurse's station. I was not a sobbing, theatrical mother begging for attention. I simply couldn't control the river that flowed from my eyes. It was involuntary and continuous.

"Mrs. Dunham," she said as she gently approached me. "Your Michael is a fine and polite young gentleman. When you are not here, he pushes other patients around in their wheelchairs and tries to help them. He is always polite to our staff. I have two sons. One is one year older than your Mike, and the other is one year younger. Their manners and behavior are just like your boy's. I can't even imagine what you are going through. Mike is your only child, isn't he?"

"Yes," I replied, "and thank you for your kind words." I can't remember her face or her name, but I will never forget her compassion. I never saw her again.

Mike later told me about his own experiences during this stay. "One time, Dr. Kim came into my room with two student nurses. I stood up out of respect to address them. All three of them lurched backwards. I could tell that they were afraid of me, so I went back to bed to lie on my side."

"Do whatever they say," other inmates told him. "If they tell you to take a shower, do it. If they tell you to eat, do it. They are watching everything that you do and writing down everything that you say."

Mike also remembers that he was given a menu to fill out for his meals each day. "Mom, I thought that they were fucking with me because no matter what I checked off, they brought me something else. I thought it was a conspiracy." I wondered if the staff collected the menus or cared what patients wanted to eat.

When I went to visit early in the day, I would go into Mike's room to observe him. It was always the same. He was quietly lying on his right side, staring, with rapid lateral eye movements.

"You can't go into patients' rooms," a nurse would exclaim as she quickly approached me. "A patient might feel cornered and threatened." Although Mike's roommate was in the bathroom, it later occurred to me that she might have meant Mike, even though he had never demonstrated any signs of violence.

With all of this going on, we had to deal with other immediate concerns. The first was that I had not told the rest of my family what was going on. The second issue was that we had not dealt with the fact that Michael couldn't return to college. We needed to get in touch with his roommates and the university. Last, the modeling and acting school kept calling me to find out why Mike had missed his last two classes. I had been avoiding these calls for as long as I could. The day of reckoning was upon us.

Chapter 12 – The Day of Reckoning

On the third day of Michael's second admission to the hospital, I knew what had to be done. We were in for the long haul, and it was now time to be proactive. My brother Jim had come to the hospital again.

"Suz, don't you think that it's time now to tell our brothers and sisters?" he asked, while maintaining their composure and kind face.

"Yes, Jim, it's time now."

I called my other five older brothers and sisters in the order of their birth. With each one, I asked, "Are you sitting down?"

"Yes."

"Michael got schizophrenia." While they all have slightly different pitches to our same common voice as siblings, they all said the exact same words.

"Oh my God, Susie, I don't know what to say." My sisters all sobbed immediately. My brothers all maintained a calm composure. Their words were all the same. "What can I do for you?"

"Pray for us." One by one, I commanded them not to tell Tommy. "His great big heart needs time to heal from his heart attack. He doesn't need any additional stress. I want you to swear to God that you won't tell him. I told you when I was ready, and I'll tell Tom when I think the time is right." They all promised. The only exception to these calls had been to my brother Mike.

"Mike, I'm lost. This problem is too large for me to handle. I'm going to have to go back to work after the end of August, or my business will fall apart and we won't be able to pay the bills. Can you come here and help me for a while?"

"Suzer, I'll come right now."

"No, Mike, wait. I need to be at home for a while. Let's wait until after Labor Day."

That part of my job was done now.

It wasn't until four months later that I told Tom. I heard a sigh and a groan in response from my little brother, who is devoutly Catholic.

"Sue, why didn't you tell me sooner? I could have been praying for Mike a lot longer." Later he told me, "On every Sunday, I pray for Mike during the consecration of The Host. It is the holiest time of the Mass."

We had to do something about the next semester of college. "Mike, can you give us a phone number for one of your college roommates? It'll take some time for you to feel better. We need to take care of the lease situation and withdraw you from classes this semester." Somehow, Mike was able to give us a phone number as he vacantly stared into space. We called his friend Jacob and explained the situation. Jacob contacted the landlord and, through fax communication, we were able to get out of our responsibilities on the lease. Jacob went on a campaign to find a replacement for Mike's space.

"Can you help the new guy with the security deposit?" was all he asked us.

"Sure we can." So we paid for the security deposit the second time, without flinching. Time had slipped away from us during this crisis, and we had waited too long to cancel Mike's classes without paying a penalty. Between the apartment and the college, the cost to cancel was $1500, and none of it meant a single thing to us. It was only money. Ironically, I thought about how every fall that Mike went back to school, I had cried. Now I was crying because he couldn't go back, and probably never would be able to.

Finally, I contacted Mrs. Augustine at the modeling and acting school. She had left me several messages asking why Mike had not attended his classes for the last two weeks. I have never been good at telling lies, so I decided to tell her that Mike had been sick.

"What's wrong?" she asked without hesitation.

"He had a nervous breakdown," I blurted out too quickly, for it hadn't been the plan to say that much. "But, we expect that he'll be better soon. Will he be able to resume his classes then?"

"What is his diagnosis?" she asked, not missing a beat.

The handwriting was on the wall. *Don't tell.* Without batting an eye, I replied that it was depression and assumed complete responsibility for Mike's present condition. "Mrs. Augustine, I think we pushed Mike too hard to go back to college. He really wants to study acting."

"As long as he doesn't have paranoid schizophrenia, that's fine. Call me back when you think that Mike is ready. We are very interested in representing him. He has a good look!"

Chapter 13 – Remembering Mike

Many have proposed that music or mathematics should be named the "universal language." I disagree. I believe that "children" should own this name as the one and only universal language. Regardless of race, religion, or national origin, all parents understand the language of loving their own child beyond comprehension. As human beings, we believe that we rule the earth and are higher forms of parents than other animals. I disagree again. Most maternal and paternal animals will risk their own lives to protect their offspring. Smaller parental animals will attack bigger predators to defend their babies. Other mammals will remove their young by the scruff of their necks, taking them from their burrows to a safe place until the danger has subsided. Still others distract the predator by running directly in front of it, but in the opposite location of the nest. In animals, we call it instinct. In humans, we call it love. Whether instinct, love, or a little of both, we all have it. As parents, we protect our children from every conceivable risk, peril, jeopardy, or threat. Sometimes we can't. Sometimes fate is determined by our genes.

On July 10th in the year 1984, I finally met my long-awaited son. He arrived eight days past his due date, after twenty-four hours of arduous labor, delivered by an emergency Cesarean section. Mike's entry to the world wasn't easy and it was ultimately my husband who saved his life, while I was helpless to get attention.

The internal monitor displayed that our baby's heart rate had dropped and remained low for much too long. The alarm sounded off for a very long time, yet no one came into our labor room.

"I'll be right back Susie," Mark quietly said, so as not to alarm me, as he left me alone in our room. He told me later how he had approached a registered nurse who was handing out breakfast trays to other new mothers on the ward. "You must come with me. Put down that tray."

"Those monitors go off all the time."

"Put down that tray! Our baby's heart rate has been down for too long! You need to come in and have a look!" He actually firmly put his hands on her elbows, directing her to stop what she was doing. She followed Mark back to our labor room and looked at the print-out, which documented my contractions and our baby's heart rate for the last five minutes. Almost immediately, she announced some sort of "code" over the intercom, and ten well-meaning professionals flipped me over onto my side, raising my right leg over the side rail to alleviate any compression on the umbilical cord. I was then rushed to the operating room and was told that our baby would be delivered soon. They increased my IV fluids and gave me oxygen on the way.

Through the hours of my labor, I had no idea what was occurring in the outside world. Apparently, a huge electrical storm had been going on all night. As the anesthesiologist began to give me a spinal anesthetic, the room darkened and out came a dozen flashlights!

"You've got to be kidding!" I said without humor. "Are you going to deliver my baby with only flashlights?" Sarcastically, I thought, *none of this looks very promising.*

The storm had knocked out the electricity in the entire hospital, but within a few minutes, the emergency generator kicked in and provided light for the surgery. At 11:33 AM, Michael was born, delivered by Cesarean, screaming loudly and apparently as healthy as we could have imagined. Mark helped the delivery nurse clean our baby up, the measure and weigh him in, just like a big fish from Lake Erie. What a catch! Michael was 21 and ½ inches long and weighed 8 pounds and 11 ounces. Soon Mark carried our baby wrapped in warmed receiving blankets to the hospital nursery. My job was now done. I was given a medication by IV that completely knocked me out and provided peaceful sleep and oblivion from the last day and night's events.

Because of the anesthetic and pain medication, it took at least twenty-four hours before I could focus my eyes well. When the nurses brought my baby to me to hold and nurse, I kept seeing two of his faces. But on the second day, I held Mike with real passion, undressed him completely, turned him over and counted all of his fingers and toes. I examined every part of him and determined independently that he was absolutely perfect in every way. He was long limbed with graceful fingers and toes. His eyes were a deep violet blue and the shock of hair that surrounded his head like a monk's was bright red. This hair later fell out and came back in so blonde that it was almost white. My attempts to nurse Mike over the previous twenty-four hours had not quieted Mike's crying, and I had given permission to give him a bottle to keep him satisfied. I fed him another supplemental bottle, burped him, and felt his downy head against my neck as he squirmed in his newborn fashion. At the age of thirty years old, my best dream and finest accomplishment had been realized. From the beginning, he was the fantasy of every little girl who has ever owned a doll, envisioning one day that she would become a real mother. Mike clung to me like any other primate baby as his father said, "Susie, he smells just like you."

Within four weeks, we had Mike baptized by Father Riley in the parish church that I had grown up in. Michael was dressed in an antique baptismal gown, which had been offered by my Aunt Jean and worn by her family members for generations. He was a lovely and perfect infant, never uttering a cry or even a whimper as the cold baptismal water was poured gently over his forehead. Father Riley offered at the end of the ceremony that he had heard that if a baby didn't cry during their baptism, it was a sign of good luck. "He's a good baby, Susie," Father Riley said at the end of the initiation of the Holy Sacrament.

Six weeks after Michael's birth, Mark and I went to our Lamaze class reunion to collectively celebrate the births of our babies. All ten sets of parents showed up with perfectly beautiful baby girls and boys, dressed in their best baby finery. It was a simple gathering, with pizza delivered to a meeting room at our local hospital, and with soft drinks available. Each couple described their own unique experiences during labor and immediately after the birth of their child. Martha, our teacher, who was a registered nurse, had prepared all of us for the very best and worst situations that might occur during labor and delivery. Our Lamaze classes had paid off big time. Martha had advised earlier, "There are ten couples in this room. Statistically, one out of ten of you will have your baby delivered by C-Section." She was absolutely right. We were apparently that statistic, but she had prepared all of us to be alert to significant complications and their symptoms during labor and delivery.

We all said goodbye to our Lamaze classmates that evening with sadness, finality, and mutual relief. All of our babies had come into the world healthy and whole.

What a delight Michael was to us! We enjoyed each and every milestone and relished in each new adventure, along with many periods of absolute terror! Many of those scary moments would eventually involve Mike's allergies, asthma, and infections, but some of the scary moments were quite ordinary.

"Mom, Mike is drinking way too much formula, and his pediatrician thinks that I should give him two heaping tablespoons of rice cereal twice a day to fill up his belly. "I'm scared Ma; I don't quite know how to do this."

"Now calm down," she said. "Here's how you do it. Don't start out with the full heaping two tablespoons in the morning! Mix just one teaspoonful into a small amount of his formula and see how he tolerates it. Put just a little on a baby spoon at the front of his mouth, on his lips. Let him work it to the back of his mouth gradually. I think that you'll be surprised. He'll like it! You should have done this a long time ago with a big baby like this!"

Mike was only six weeks old and I was almost immobilized by the fear of this experiment, but I proceeded just as my mother had told me. The first little spoonful was met with interest from my roly-poly infant. He did exactly what my mother had told me. He moved it around in his mouth and gradually swallowed it.

"Ooh-la, ooh-la, ooh-la," he screamed.

I figured out that this was infant talk for "more." Boldly, I prepared the prescribed two tablespoons of cereal mixed with formula and fed him the rest. I couldn't feed him fast enough! Finally, after I delivered the last small teaspoonful on his baby spoon, I saw his eyes slam shut. It was as if I had put a club to his head! I then called my mother on the phone, long-distance, and reported to her that my mission had been accomplished.

"He loved it, Mom. He's out like a light and I can't even wake him up even when I am burping him."

"That's the point, Susie. Now go take a nap yourself. You're tired!"

How totally sweet Mike was, right from the start! He smiled and "cooed" early, and was utterly charming to both of us. The first six months were filled with the usual baby events, such as round-the-clock feedings, diaper changing, food introductions, and colic. Mike's entry into our world was a life-changing experience, but we tried to handle it responsibly. We worked opposite shifts so that at least one parent would be with Mike most of the time. Those were the days of no sleep, time, or money. In spite of how tough it all was, we were smitten with Mike's gummy smile and crinkled-up, mirthful eyes.

By the time he was nine months old, we began the "my baby" game. I would greet Mark at the door and give him a quick kiss, with Mike on my hip. Mark would kiss Mike too. Then, I would pat Mike and tell Mark, "This is MY baby!"

Mark would pretend to wrestle Mike from my arms and say, "No, no, he's MY baby!" This game would go on and on many times as we "struggled" to get "my baby" back in each of our own arms. This game went on for at least another year or two, and it was always met with hilarious laughter from Mike. He was never confused by our silly act, but enjoyed being the center of attention.

I remember the days when Mike was still in his walker, and chased me at rapid speed down the hallway of our apartment when the buzzer on the dryer rang to declare that the load was done. Later, as he began to walk, he would cling to my then-strong leg at the hip as I walked that same hallway to answer the door of our apartment when the doorbell rang.

"Forgive me, please, for taking so long to answer the door," I said, "As you can see, I have this huge growth on my right leg."

We were on a very strict budget for food, formula, and baby diapers the first two years of Mike's life, which left very little extra for luxuries of any kind. But Mark was a genius at collecting and hoarding loose change. Sometimes, on Fridays, a miracle would happen.

He would say, "Let's pack Mike up and go to Krogers." I knew what Mark was up to. There was a mechanical bouncing horse at the front door, which ate up one quarter at a time. Krogers was often our destination on a Friday night. We had to hold on to Mike while he got bounced slightly back and forth and up and down, as the mechanical horse simulated galloping.

Mark would report when the rides were finished, "I still have some money left for a pizza."

"Wow! Where did that come from?" I'd ask with admiration.

No one but my husband, who woke me up from a sound sleep at 7:00 in the morning and insisted that I crawl quietly behind him down the short hall to peer into Mike's room would have ever believed what we heard and saw. Mike was only thirteen months old, but he pointed to a 99-cent multicolored rubber ball that Mark had bought for him on a whim the previous day.

"It's a pwetty ball. It's a weally, weally, pwetty ball!" he said in an "Elmer Fudd" voice as he stood upright in his crib. Mike had been saying many words for months, but a complete sentence coming out of a baby who was just thirteen months old wasn't something that either one of us could have expected.

Mike's language skills were exceptional, and he was also a genuine clown. When he was eighteen months, we would ask him to say multi-syllabic words. Mike would parrot them as we fell down on the floor in hilarious laughter. "Say delicious, Mike." "Say Mississippi, Mike." "Say unbelievable." "Say incomprehensible, Mike." The list would go on and on along with the rolling around and the raucous laughter that Mark and I displayed. Mike would say the words and then cover his own face with his hands as he laughed at his own antics after each performance. We only stopped when he tired of his accomplishments, pointed at us, and boldly announced, "No!" Usually it was bedtime.

Saturday mornings were sometimes glorious for me. Mark, always an early riser, got up with Mike and made him homemade pancakes or waffles, allowing me to sleep in for a couple of hours. Mike was about two years old when we began buying Disney tapes, and soon we had most of them. "Sleeping Beauty" was one of our first purchases. Once Mark was worn out from breakfast and the early-day demands of our toddler, he told Mike, "Why don't you go and wake up Sleeping Beauty?" Now, of course, Mike had been previously told, "Let Mom sleep." In something of a semi-sleep condition, I had heard all of it. The gates were opened, I realized, as my toddler jumped on top of me and woke me up completely with a huge grin and a big snotty kiss.

"Wake up Sweeping Beauty!"

I couldn't help but laugh as I wiped his snot from my face. "Ugh! Mike, your nose is all snotty! Go get me a Kleenex." Of course, he always ran away when I offered to wipe his nose because it was always sore from continuous wiping.

The days went on and on with the same mundane tasks, and why I happen to have this specific memory, which isn't documented in photos, is beyond me. I remember taking warm towels out of the dryer and throwing them on the bed or sofa so that I could fold them. Mike was my constant companion and was always into something. Early on, he dived into my pile of warm dried clothes and rolled around in them like a puppy, relishing in their radiant warmth. This game went on for years and later, as his verbal skills increased, he asked, "Mom, can I roll around in the warm towels?" Then, I simply invited him, throwing them on top of him, but always cautioning that once they were folded, we were done with this fun. Looking back, I must have understood that housework and child-raising were not mutually exclusive jobs.

By the age of three, Mike was speaking in complete and clear sentences, using adjectives and adverbs correctly. On my mother's 70th birthday, he looked like Tom Thumb, dressed in his red plaid knickers with matching bow tie, suspenders, crisp white shirt, white knee socks, and saddle shoes. All eight of us siblings gathered to surprise our mother and celebrate the day. My sister Nan had come the farthest, from Arizona, and hadn't seen Mike since he was a baby. I had picked Mike up and placed him on a chair so that he could see what was going on in the dining room of my mother's hundred-year-old house. Even at three years old, his world wasn't only about himself. He knew what was going on with other people and reached out to them.

He had a deep little voice and asked questions that were much more appropriate to adults. "Hello, Aunt Nan. How are you? It's so very nice to see you! Today is Grandma Katy's birthday. We all surprised her!" My big sister swept Mike into her arms, and hugged and kissed him, just as she had done with me as a child.

"Susie, he's so smart and cute! He looks and acts just like you did when you were little!"

The old homestead was filled with our huge family and tons of mother's friends, who all considered her their "best friend." That was simply who she was—everyone's best friend. Mom always had a ready ear for anybody's problems and an open pocketbook in time of need. I looked around our old house, loving every minute that I spent with my family. There was Mom, cutting her large birthday cake iced in white frosting with eight green shamrocks representing her children, all bordering the words, "Happy 70th Birthday Mom".

I remembered the day that I had presented Mike to my mother and had asked, "Mom, isn't he the most beautiful baby you have ever seen?" I caught her entirely off guard with this question, which provoked a response that I had not anticipated.

"Susie, first of all, I have many grandchildren, and I love them all. There are no favorites. Also, I just happen to think that my babies were the most beautiful babies that were ever born! But he does look exactly like one of my own babies." That fact changed things. My mother couldn't help herself and doted on Mike as long as she lived. Mom would call to announce that I should expect a UPS package for Mike, at least four times a year. Inside were cheap but clever little toys that any little boy would adore.

My father had been gone for a number of years. The upkeep of our large turn of the century house had become more of a burden for her than a joy to own. At seventy years old, she decided to start over. With both sadness and relief, she sold the old house and moved to Indianapolis to live with my sister Kathy and be close to my brother Mike, who was everyone's hero. Mom felt safe with them in her older years, but every summer, she came to stay with us for two months. She washed our clothes, performed extraordinary small acts of kindness on a daily basis, and somehow dispelled any notion that we had a burden with Mike's fragile health. There was always a feeling of confidence that everything would be all right as long as Mom was around. Each and every day, she took Mike out to eat at the restaurant of his choice and played with him endlessly on the floor with his toys. Mother died when Mike was fifteen years old. I'm glad she didn't live to see what happened to him.

Mike must have been three and a half when I became absolutely certain that he was a genius. After fixing him lunch and cleaning up the kitchen, I heard him ask with complete sincerity, "Mom, will you do me a favor?"

"Of course, Mike. What?"

"Will you just agree with anything that I say?" Of course I agreed as I tried to contain my snickering. I understood right then and there that he already knew what all big boys want. *Feed me when I am hungry and don't disagree with my opinions.*

We didn't just play with Mike. He was in charge and often initiated exactly how he wanted us to play. If we were quietly watching television and not paying enough attention to him, he would stand directly in front of us with a huge grin on his face. "Whatever you do, don't tickle me!" he commanded as he lifted up his shirt, exposing his chubby little belly. He already understood reverse psychology.

Mike must have been about five years old when he boldly announced to us that he would like to have a butler. "Why do you want a butler Mike? You already have one and his name is Dad." It was true. If Mike wanted anything special, such as popcorn, a milkshake, or ice cream, his father served it to him with great pleasure and aplomb at his table and chair set.

One of my favorite memories involves Mike's first grade. We were lucky to have a newly graduated, first-year teacher, Mrs. Mooney. I can't exactly say why she took such a special liking to Mike. I only know that she apparently adored him. During the first week of school, she established the duties of the "line leader." One person from each row had special responsibilities for one week. He/she collected and handed out papers, helped with the blackboard and chalk, and was the leader of his or her own row. This position made a first-grader a certified "big shot." Mike was chosen the very first day to master the world of Row One of Mrs. Mooney's first-grade classroom. On Friday, his responsibilities weren't quite over. Mike had to choose the next big-shot.

I awaited the school bus to find out how Mike's day had gone, knowing that he had to pass his crown on to someone else. "Mike, certainly you picked Danny, your good friend, to be the next line leader, didn't you?"

"No, Mom. I picked this Indian boy that nobody likes."

"Wow, Mike. That was nice. Why did you do that?"

"Mom, I wanted him to feel important."

The memory of this incident has caused me to cry with joy and pride many times. At the age of six, Mike had defined his own persona. He understood the pain of others.

The memories of those early years almost blend together like a casserole in my mind. It always seemed that the "New Year" began in the summer because the cold months of winter in the Midwest were often so harsh. Mike was a "water baby" from the age of one, swimming in Lake Erie with his grandpa and dad, riding on grandpa's back as he swam underwater. I have the most incredible memory of Mike at the age of two, holding hands with his paternal grandparents as they walked the short distance to our neighborhood beach. It was a windy day, and the waves rolled onto the beach mighty and high as they broke on the shoreline. Over and over, Mike ran fearlessly along the shoreline, throwing himself into the huge waves. Over and over, he would recover his footing in the shallow water, coming out each time coughing, spitting out sand and crying. But then, once composed, he would do it again! Mike was born with absolutely no fear of water and natural buoyancy. Later, he became a very strong swimmer. Our summers always involved a huge celebration on the 4th of July with Mike, from the age of two, holding a sparkler under supervision. Each year, on July 10th, Mike's birthday, our celebration was something special, taking Mike's friends to restaurants, water parks, and amusement places. Summers were always glorious.

My memories have survived after many years of cutting up pumpkins for Halloween, then deciding whose turn it was to take Mike trick-or-treating and who stayed home to hand out the treats. Eventually Mike went with his buddies. Thanksgivings were shared with both sides of our family, always with travel attached. Christmases involved our own made-up rituals of getting up at 6:00 AM, opening presents, going to Mass, then driving a distance to share the day with Mark's family. Easters were celebrated with Dad hiding the eggs, which we had all colored together the day before, along with hiding the Easter basket and small trinkets that the Easter Bunny had left. The Tooth Fairy visited when necessary and left a silver dollar under Mike's pillow each time he lost a tooth.

There were many family events, vacations to faraway places, and short jaunts. I can't even remember all the trips to zoos, snow skiing, toboggan runs, amusement parks, festivals, and cultural events. I simply remember that we all enjoyed them together. How could I sum up the long list of wonderful memories that we have of our boy? In the beginning, he was our perfect little baby doll, later our little "Buddy" and playmate. As Mike matured, we considered him a fair and honored equal. Somehow we had been spared from tragedy through all the years of our son learning to cross the street, riding his bicycle, and climbing tall trees. The three of us had enjoyed a symbiotic relationship, with all three of us giving and taking and enjoying the ride. The "ride" certainly hadn't always been easy, but there had been many supreme moments of joy in our lives.

Mike's asthma, allergies, and infections had always been a huge challenge to control, but during Mike's middle-school years, a new hurdle presented itself. Mike began to suffer from rapid onset and dramatic episodes of asthma as a result of acid reflux. Some people might experience "heartburn" when stomach acid gets into their esophagus, but when even a small amount of stomach acid enters the lungs, the results can be severe and terrifying. Mark and I found ourselves forced to make some decisions that were life-changing as Mike's episodes increased in frequency. Both of us were missing work, and Mike was missing school. It was time to regroup and decide exactly what was most important, and of course Mike's health was at the top of our list.

We decided to build a totally "green" house, on Lake Erie next door to Mark's parents. This environment was cleaner than in the city. We had the support of Mark's parents, retired high school teachers, who helped us to home-school Mike until his symptoms subsided. We knew that he had become a little chubby in his middle-school years, but had been advised by his allergist that as Mike grew taller, so would his esophagus, and that eventually, he would "out-grow" this new problem. Thanks to Mark's parents' commitment we were able to go forward. As a team, we challenged Mike daily with lessons that were much more difficult than he would ever encounter in public school. Mike returned to the public school system, enrolled in a college prep curriculum, and excelled academically. He graduated in the top ten of the males in his class after taking advanced placement courses in all subjects during his senior year.

Mike took his first summer job at the age of fourteen, working in an ice-cream store, baking the cones and hand-dipping ice cream for the customers. He wanted to take scuba-diving lessons and buy his own gear. We had to drive him to and from this job and almost gagged at how sickeningly sweet he smelled when we picked him up. The following three summers, he worked as a busboy in a fancy restaurant, earning huge tips because all of the waitresses thought that he was such a hard worker. The next two summers, Mike worked at a local country club as a dock boy. Once again, he reaped the benefits of his hard work and good people skills. Mike was born with good manners, but quickly learned the diplomacy necessary to handle the demands of the very rich.

In the year 2002, Mike graduated from high school and we happily shipped him off to college. By this time, he was a somewhat mature, grownup young man. Once in a while, he showed up quite unexpectedly on a Friday afternoon. He often parked his car next door at his grandparents' so as not to bring attention to his arrival. Quietly, he would enter the front door and secretly slip up the stairs to surprise me as I washed clothes or emptied the dishwasher. I never saw him coming as he would sneak up behind me, grab me, and bend me over backwards, planting a huge kiss on my mouth.

"Mother, I'm hungry. Make me some food!"

Other times, he sneaked up the stairs, finding me unaware, picked me up from behind, and twirled me around! My playmate was now much bigger than I was, but still my delightful companion.

"Mom, I need help with my wash." After the usual initial shock, I would laugh.

"OK Mike, bring it up here to the laundry room. I'll do it."

Sometimes I became impatient and asked, "Don't you think that it's time that you learned to do your own wash, Mike?"

"Mom," Mike would hilariously laugh and say, "You may be little, but you're like Sea Biscuit, the race horse. You can do anything!" It never occurred to him that I was getting older and running out of steam. But he was so full of life and fun that there was nothing I could deny him.

For all of Mike's life, we had enjoyed a playful relationship. While I certainly took care of his basic needs, I had been a much better "big kid" than a mother. It was Mark who had insisted upon routine and structure in our home. This was a good thing because I simply wasn't capable of setting up rules and following through.

Mike and I had shared hundreds of "hellos" and "goodbyes" with a hug and kiss, followed by our usual silly banter.

"You're my baby!"

"You're my mammy!"

But not on this day in August of the year 2005, when I entered his room in the psychiatric unit he had been admitted to for the second time, and called his name with no response. Mike was in a severely catatonic state, lying motionless on his side, except for the rapid lateral movements of his eyes. I looked on in horror and thought, *He looks exactly like the patients that I cared for years ago, who were brain injured at birth or had traumatic head injuries.* Mike's brain injury was just as real but simply of a different nature. This was no ordinary bad dream. It was a virtual nightmare of the most dreaded kind.

My mind was flooded with over twenty-one years of memories on that hot summer day. I remembered who Mike was as a person, and specifically, who he was and what he meant to me, as I flagged his psychiatrist who was there on rounds. I asked for a few minutes of his time, in private. Dr. Kim looked tired, but conceded. I broke down and sobbed. Dr. Kim told me that the staff all knew that Mike was a fine gentleman. He told me that what had happened was sad. I knew at that very moment that we were truly in very serious trouble. Doctors don't use the word "sad" unless they really mean it.

"Will Mike ever be the same, Dr. Kim?"

"No. He will never be the same again."

Chapter 14 – Discharged Again

Mike understood that he was coming home and waited quietly for his discharge papers to be processed. He had been prescribed Abilify, in the lowest therapeutic dose, to control his psychotic symptoms. He was quiet and subdued while waiting with me to accomplish the signing of his discharge documents. He looked totally "geeked out" to me, with eyes that were wide and not comprehending all that was going on around him. *His brains are scrambled*, I thought with deep sadness.

Another young man approached the nurses' station. He appeared to be in his early thirties, quite cute and very amiable. "He has what I have," he said, as he smiled at me.

"Really, what do you have?"

"Paranoid schizophrenia. My mother knows when I am having problems because I get angry and start pointing at the ground. My psychiatrist tried to wean me off my medication after I lost my job and benefits."

"That's too bad. You look very healthy to me right now. It was nice of you to talk with us." He then described what he thought about the other male patients on the ward.

"Most of the guys are OK, but you have to watch out for that one." He was directing his eyes towards Mike's roommate. I wished him well and told him that Mike was going home today. He mentioned that all of the patients liked Mike and thought that he was a good kid who tried to be nice to everyone.

The same nurse discharged Mike as before with almost the same instructions, except this time she discussed Mike's other new prescription, Ativan, a sedative. "Don't be afraid to use this if Mike becomes anxious," she advised. This seemed a peculiar instruction because to my knowledge, it had never been given in the hospital.

Why hadn't they given this to Mike when he was assaulted by the devils? I looked at Mike. He smelled bad and his hair was greasy. *Why hadn't they supervised a shower? How could they let him get into this smelly condition?*

We walked out together with a large bag of clean clothes that had never been worn. "Mike, when we get home, the first thing that you are going to do is get into the bathtub."

"I am going to fill up the bathtub and let you soak," I told Mike upon our arrival home. "Take your clothes off when the tub is full."

Mike protested, "Mom, I am a grown man. I can't be naked in front of you."

"That is perfectly fine. Put this hand towel over your private parts. I'll wash your hair, back, and under your arms, and you can do the rest. It's certainly not the first time that I bathed a grown man, Mike." The mission was accomplished just in time. My brother Mike and sister Kathy showed up at our front door, after a five-hour drive.

"Kathy, would you like to shave Mike?" I offered her this task because I knew that she wanted to be helpful. She was a nurse. It would make her feel better if she did something nice for Mike. Then I told Mike to brush his teeth. After the discharge and personal hygiene experience, Mike was absolutely exhausted. He gratefully went to his own bed, and I had time to talk with my siblings.

"He's a lot better now," I told my brother Mike. I saw the "bullet look" in my brother's eyes, a family trait we show when any of us is surprised or alarmed. He must have wondered, *what was it like before?* I could see the look of shock in my brother's eyes, but proceeded. "Michael, I can't tell you, how much I appreciate that Kathy and you came to see Mike. Also, I am so glad that you are planning to help me out when I go back to work. Let me get past Labor Day. I'll stay at home until then. Mike, are you sure that you want to do this?" My brother looked directly into my eyes and soul. I will never forget the words he answered.

"I will come whenever you tell me to come. I am retired now. Suzer, there is nothing that would give me greater pleasure than to help you. I'll come each week and let you get back to work, and I'll stay as long as it takes."

"Mike, it might take a long time. Maybe Mike will never get better."

"He will," my brother replied with confidence.

Kathy and Mike had always been close. They were next to each other in birth order. Kathy was ten and Mike eleven when I was born. They had both attended the same Catholic elementary school. For years, I had heard the stories about how they had taken me on a sled as a baby while they sold Christmas cards. They were also helping our mother, who had her hands quite full with duties, by baby-sitting me, as they went on their mission. They claimed that it was my sunny disposition that won the hearts of their "customers." Jokingly, they had also told me that I was a perfect "prop" in my purple, hand-knitted snow suit, as they became first-class salesmen in the world of Christmas cards. "You never cried, Susie."

Now it was my turn to cry. "Michael, how could it be that we only left Mike for five days and that this happened?" I put my face in my hands and sobbed.

"Susie, it always happens that way. I have friends at my club. They left for work in the morning and when they came home that evening, their son was the same as Mike. It happened that fast." My brother cracked open beers for the three of us. There was a lot of quiet talk as we waited for Mark to come home. After a couple hours, Mike came out of his bedroom and we all walked to the neighborhood beach together to watch the waves for just a few minutes.

In spite of the fact that our Michael was blurry-eyed and not comprehending what was going on, he said, "Thanks Aunt Kathy and Uncle Mike. I'm glad that you came to see me." Then he went quietly back to bed.

My brother Mike looked into the refrigerator and threw together a meal. This was just the first of many acts of kindness that he would provide.

Chapter 15 – My Brother Michael

After Labor Day and through the months of September, October, and most of November, my brother Mike drove five hours back and forth from Indianapolis to stay with our son so that we could go to work. He usually arrived on Sunday night and went home on Friday, after I had returned from my sales calls. He cleaned our house, shopped for food, cooked our meals, washed our clothes, folded them and put them away. He even cut the grass each week and brought in the mail. He made it possible for us to earn a living and to be only concerned with our son once we were home. He took care of all of the other details. My beautiful brother Michael saved our family in every conceivable way.

He quickly caught on that it was important to speak to Mike in a soft, calm, and reassuring voice, as Mike couldn't tolerate loud noises and often didn't understand anything but short, direct sentences. Brother Mike was the one true witness of the real suffering involved in Mike's disease. Each night, he brought out the beers and let me cry. At first, once our Mike was in bed, my crying came in a quiet stream of silent, steady tears. Then came the sobbing that only occurs with real grief and true rage.

"I want to scream, Mike."

"Suz, I know a place out in the country. I can take you there and you can scream as loud as you want." It was only the exhaustion of this exercise that made me decline his offer. Later, each evening, my brother served me a plate of food which I had refused to eat earlier. He put small portions on my plate and urged me to eat "just a little."

Each week, my brother and I took Mike to see Dr. Kim. Gradually, Mike's dose of Abilify was increased, 2.5 or 5 mg at a time, until we could quiet the voices that tormented him day and night. By November, they were indeed silent, but at what cost! The side-effects of the drugs were as bizarre and varied as the disease itself.

In the beginning, Mike displayed terrible tremors in his hands, especially his right hand. The most bizarre and heart-wrenching symptoms were akathisia and akinesia. With akathisia, Mike had the inability to sit down, and had feelings of restlessness and the constant need to keep moving. Mike went from chair to sofa, then to the loveseat, then from one bed to another, often covering himself with a pile of blankets – and then repeated all of the above.

Sometimes he stood directly in front of a chair, got halfway down to sit, and then stopped in mid-air, suspended in space and time. It seemed to take an eternity for him to finally sit down. "Aren't you going to sit down, Mike?" I would ask.

"Yes, that was what I was doing." This must have been a new symptom of his catatonia.

I wondered about the source of his restlessness. Mike would touch his chest at his heart and say, "It burns." Much later, when Mike was able to describe his continuous torment, he said, "It felt as if there was a steady current of electricity flowing through my body. It was very uncomfortable." Since then, I have read others' descriptions of this bizarre side-effect of anti-psychotic medications. Some describe it as a feeling of "electro-cution."

On September 19, 2005, we were invited to share a birthday cake with Mike's paternal uncle, who lives across the street. "Mike, can you take a quick shower, brush your teeth, and put on some clean clothes?" I asked. "Let's go across the street for a quick piece of cake." Mike had not showered for a couple of days and followed my advice. I stood in the foyer and looked at my handsome son as he descended the stairs in clean khakis and a knit collared shirt. "You look like a million bucks, Mike! Give your mom a big smile." With that, Mike attempted to smile at me, but what I saw was ghoulish. He had absolutely no control over his facial muscles and what I observed was a distorted grimace. This new side-effect, *akinesia*, which is complete or partial loss of muscle movement, was such a shock to me that I felt my stomach fall and thought that I was going to vomit on the spot.

I thought that I had seen it all, but there was more to come. Then came the open gaping mouth, with Mike's thick tongue in sight, but somehow retracted. The constant drooling began, with saliva running out of both sides of his mouth in a steady stream. Here was my son, a champion among men, drooling non-stop.

Each time that Mike's Abilify was increased, another side-effect surfaced. Then he began to have trouble swallowing. While all of the previously mentioned side-effects were devastating to watch, this one, which remained with Mike for well over two years, was quite frightening. I was certain that he would choke on his food as I watched him at mealtimes.

With each increase, Mike lay in his bed and described that a painful clamp had been put on his brain. Standing up quickly would make Mike feel as if he might faint. The drug caused postural hypotension, which is low blood pressure, upon standing. It became clear that he had lost the ability to control his body temperature, and we constantly worried that he might die quite suddenly from a heat stroke. Antipsychotics also have this unusual side-effect.

We kept Dr. Kim informed of Mike's behaviors and increased side-effects of the drug. He prescribed a drug called Cogentin, which is also used for Parkinson's Disease, to alleviate the side-effects from Mike's antipsychotic medication. This drug was also increased gradually over time, and it took the maximum dose to stop the ghoulish side-effects. But this miracle drug came along with its own side-effects. Mike's pupils became so dilated that he developed an extreme sensitivity to light. The drooling finally stopped, only to be replaced with an extremely dry mouth that enhanced Mike's continuous difficulty with swallowing food. As Mike came back to reality, he wryly said, "Uncle Mike, this is the disease that keeps on giving."

I know that Mike talked with his uncle about suicide. These were private conversations between the two of them. Somehow my brother talked him out of it one day or one moment at a time. Statistically, 15% of people who develop schizophrenia die, mostly by suicide. Michael understood the gravity of his illness, mourned his loss of functioning, and suffered profoundly from the side-effects of his medications. My beautiful brother Mike gave him the encouragement to continue and told him repeatedly, "You will get better."

My brother had helped every single member of our family over the years, in one way or another. It might have been with money, a service, time or understanding. He gave us the greatest gift of all. Single-handedly, he preserved the life of our only child, as we tried to survive and lick our fresh wounds.

Chapter 16 – Ninety Days and Nights

For ninety days and ninety nights, our home was a virtual hell. Nothing in my years of nursing had prepared me for the true suffering that I witnessed as my child came out of his world of torment. The voices were there 24/7. They asked him questions over and over. They accused him of sins that he had never committed. They were threatening, accusing, and mocking. Sometimes there was just one, sometimes two or three were present, and held a continual dialogue regarding exactly how they were going to kill him. Sometimes there were many, meaning hundreds, in cacophony. Later, after the "good" voices turned mean and cruel, I asked Mike, "Were they ever kind again?"

"Sometimes," Mike replied, "as they described exactly how they were going to burst a blood vessel in my brain, they would tell me not to worry because it would be over soon."

The continuous onslaught of horrendous medication side-effects made his journey back all the more unbearable to watch. Ah, this disease was an incredible invention of no less than the devil himself. Between the disease and the drugs, his condition mimicked almost all other diseases in one way or another.

My phone rang many times a day. My loving family not only worried about Michael, but feared for my own sanity. They desperately wanted to hear some good news. How could I explain that there wasn't any? How could I accurately describe what was happening? Then the unsolicited advice began to come. For my six older siblings, I was the treasured baby girl they had raised along with our parents. They took ownership as parental figures and also expected obedience from me.

"Susie, you need to get some medicine to calm you down and allow you to cope with this."

"Suz, you need to lay off the beer. It's a depressant and will only make things worse. We know that you're crying all the time."

"Susie, you need to apply for Social Security right now. It'll take a long time to get it."

I wasn't ready or willing to hear any of these things and, after a while, made one of the most difficult decisions I have ever made in my life. I asked my brother Mike to shut down the phones from family. "Michael, Jim did it for me in business for a while and it helped. Tell them that I love them, but don't have the will at this time to discuss my own welfare or any future plans for Mike. Tell them that I'll call them when I want to talk to them. They can't possibly know what is going on here. Ask them to pray and just send cards."

"It'll be done tomorrow," my brother Mike replied. "I'll tell them to ask me or Jim for news. I came here to take instructions, not to give them." This truth gave me the freedom to go to work. My brother would take care of Mike and follow my instructions exactly. He understood that I had always been compulsively organized and a planner. In spite of the fact that almost nothing was under my control, he had the spiritual wisdom and the genius to provide the illusion. With Jim's and Mike's intervention, my phones suddenly became silent again.

Even though I had broken some hearts with my distance, the cards, letters, and prayers came. My sister Nan began sending cards and long letters to Mike almost every other day. Finally, I broke my silence and called her.

"Nan, I appreciate the cards and letters, but Mike can't read anymore. Just send a card with a brief note, once a week."

"What do you mean that he can't read anymore?"

"Nan, he has cognitive and expressive aphasia. He doesn't always understand what we're saying unless the statement is simple and short. I asked him to read a short sentence the other day and he couldn't." I tried to explain further. "Mike read the words and said them aloud."

Mike told me, "Mother, I can say the words, but I don't know what the fuck they mean."

"Nan, it's like a stroke in many ways. It's like he had a head injury and can't remember or understand anything."

"I'll just send cards with a short message," she kindly replied, as she cried for us long-distance from Arizona. Then the cards kept coming.

My brother Joe, a bona-fide genius, who studied with the Jesuit priests, sent Mike a colorful, kind, and sweetly amusing letter. "Mike, you got kicked in the head, but in time, you'll be OK." He later came to visit Mike in November and spoke to Mike with the same natural respect he always had. There had always been a certain affinity between Mike and his Uncle Joe. Besides affection, there existed a mutual respect for raw intelligence.

I spoke with Jim on most days regarding Mike and business. He told me that he cried every day and that Frances and Kathy were having trouble sleeping. "When will you tell Tommy?" He was trying to tell me in a quiet, gentlemanly way that I needed to talk to all our siblings, and that they too were grieving. I listened to what he was proposing with a deaf ear. I was no longer the sweet little girl that they all remembered. I was angry, hurt, and in no mood to be obedient to anyone's advice.

I remembered the awful day Moxie died. Moxie had been our beloved dog for eleven years but had a terrible habit of chasing cars. Moxie was absolutely homely, but the smartest and kindest dog that we had ever owned. He had the coat, head, and tail of a Labrador retriever, along with the legs and body of a Dachshund. Mother had his tail "docked" to match his short body when he was just a puppy. Moxie would "talk" groaning and yowling and yawning whenever asked. He shook hands and did tricks that only mongrels are smart enough to learn. It was our opinion that most thoroughbreds had all the brains bred out of them. Moxie was Dad's constant companion whenever he was home from work. When Dad was home, Moxie belonged only to him, staring at him with worshipful eyes. It was a good thing that Dad wasn't home on the fateful day that Moxie met his demise. Mom, Tommy and I, all saw it happen. If the car hadn't tried to stop, Moxie might have dodged his death once again. But instead, he rolled under the car and caught the right rear tire after escaping the left front. Tom was only twelve years old and ran to comfort our wounded and dying pet. Moxie bit him, right before dying.

It was something like that for me. I had absolutely no patience for advice, ignorance, or confusion about this no-fault brain disease. After Mike's illness, almost all of my kind virtues vanished. I was something like Moxie. I wondered, *Why don't you understand that the wounded bite?*

Mike's three best friends came to visit one by one. Evan, who had been Mike's best friend in high school, was the first to come, some time in early September.

"All us guys miss you," said Evan, trying to make conversation.

Mike stared off into the distance and after what seemed an eternity asked, "Did you take care of my problem with the apartment lease?"

"Yes, Jacob found someone to come in with us and take over your share of the lease." Mike continued to stare vacantly for what seemed to be a very long time.

"Thank you for coming to see me, Evan. I'm tired now." Mike went back to his room to lie down. I could see that Evan was terribly shaken. He was the first person outside of family that we had allowed to visit with Mike. Evan began to cry.

"I didn't realize that he was this sick."

"Evan, thank you for coming to see Mike, but I have one question. Was Mike OK during the fall semester?"

"Yes, he was fine all of the first semester. It was in later January that we saw a change."

"Thank you, Evan. That makes perfect sense to me now. That's when I think that the change started."

I hugged Evan goodbye. Whether I believed it myself or not, I told him, "He'll get better. It's just going to take some time."

David came next, later in September. He'd been Mike's first best friend. He lived down the street from us, in the old days, in the city. From the time when Mike was two and David was four, they were inseparable. Many childhood adventures took place on our quiet little street, and I had been part of some of their misadventures. I remembered the huge bush that grew at the back of our property. Mike and David had somehow rigged up their own bungee-cord device and asked me to try it! They pulled down and tied the branches to an elastic tether, and then rapidly released the bungee cord. At 39 years old, I had gone flying into the air! It had always been that way with David. He had been an exciting friend. David was in the Air Force and overseas when I'd called his mother to tell her that Mike had become ill.

"Oh my God, Susie, I don't know what to say. I'll email David right away. We'll pray for you." I was so appreciative. Betty had been a wonderful friend and neighbor to me as well.

David returned from overseas and came to see Mike the very next day. He came armed with light-hearted stories about his layover in Scotland and his adventures with all the pretty Scottish girls. He patiently showed Mike his photos on our computer and carefully ignored Mike's constant drooling. He spoke to Mike like a man and ignored his present infirmity. This was the first day that Mike had stayed out of bed for more than two hours at a time, but eventually tired. David said goodbye to him in a "man-to-man" fashion; then watched as Mike ascended the stairs to return to his room. I hugged and kissed David as I thanked him for lifting our spirits. David did not cry.

"Mike will get better," he told me. "He won't settle for anything less."

Thanksgiving break came and Mike's third best friend, Casey, announced that he would come to visit for a couple days. We had a unique relationship with Casey and his parents. Don and Melissa, Casey's parents, had grown up spending summers at Peach Tree Beach in their parents' cottages. They were the "summer neighbors" and both played with my husband as children. Later, they grew up, married, and remained our friends. Eventually, when we spent summers at the lake, our children became friends and shared their own summer adventures for many years.

Mark and I owned a small summer cottage for a while and one day, Casey showed up asking for Michael.

"I'm going down to the lagoon to go fishing," he announced in his squeaky little seven-year-old voice. "Can Michael come with me?" I looked carefully at Casey and his get-up. He wore a sweatshirt, sweat pants, a life preserver, and rubber boots. Proudly, he showed us his Fisher-Price fishing pole and tackle box. Melissa and Don had two older children, so I was certain that they knew what they were doing. Was it really OK to send my seven-year-old down to the lagoon to fish without my supervision? Well, Melissa was a veteran mother and she thought it was OK, so it must be! I took direction, garbed Mike exactly the same, and boldly sent him on his way to a new adventure.

"Melissa, you were my inspiration," I later told her, "for what was appropriate here at the lake, but I walked down to the lagoon to spy on our boys every half hour."

"I must have been there in between!" she added with a laugh. Ah, the freedom we gave those little boys was only exceeded by their proud bucket of inedible bottom-feeding fish.

For years, we had brought David along with us to Peach Tree Beach, sharing with Casey's parents the "summer beach experience." As we pulled our red Radio Flyer wagon along with us, which carried our cooler full of bologna sandwiches, chips, and Kool-Aid, we looked forward to another happy day. There we stayed for hours, combating sunburn with heavy-duty sunscreen as we watched our children exhaust themselves in the rolling waves. Everyone slept well at night, after an exhaustive search for fireflies caught in simple glass jars, and a burger, corn on the cob, and watermelon in their bellies. Life had been so simple in those days.

Our boys grew up, one year at a time, and later had their own wild experiences of chasing down fourteen-year-old girls to kiss. Our friendship continued as our children ventured into high school. Then the experiences of their college years kept us tied together. When Casey came to see Michael on his Thanksgiving break, it was a continuum. Casey had always been a real gem and comic delight since childhood, and this visit was no different, but for one exception – Mike was sick. He brought his usual ray of sunshine to our home with stories of his college antics, and Mike was grateful for his visit. Somehow, it was a normalizing factor. Then it was time for Casey to leave. Michael was exhausted, said his goodbyes and made his escape to bed. I walked Casey to the door and as with the others, hugged and kissed him goodbye as I thanked him for coming to see Mike. This time, the goodbye was different as Casey broke into loud sobs.

"Mrs. Dunham, I was there with Mike on the night that you and Mr. Dunham left on vacation. Mike and I drove your boat out into the lake and went swimming. Then we went to Put-in-Bay and had a couple beers and a pizza. Mike looked happy, and there was nothing wrong. We came home and I went back to our cottage. The next day, Michael didn't want to do anything and then later, he wouldn't answer his phone. I didn't worry. You know how Michael's always been. Even as kids, he would go out with the rest of us for hours, but at some point, he needed to get away for a while and have his quiet time, just for an hour or so." I understood this completely as I remembered the howling fights that his toy dinosaurs had with each other in the quiet of his room with the door closed. "Mrs. Dunham, Mike's an only kid. He needed that time to re-group. He always came back for more fun with the rest of us, when he was ready. I thought it was like that, only he didn't come back out this time. I feel so bad that my best friend had his mind playing tricks on him, while I was out having a good time."

"Don't think twice about it Casey. We all missed it."

Each day out on the road was both difficult and reinforcing.

"How is Mike? We are praying for him." Many of my customers noticed after a time that I had lost close to twenty pounds and wanted to feed me snacks or take me to lunch.

"Thank you, but I have to stay on track and get home."

My in-laws had suddenly become old. This was an additional sadness for me as I understood how helpful and generous they had always been. In spite of their age, they took over in Mark's and my absences, after my brother Mike left. Each day, they would plan to play cards with Mike and often took Mike out to lunch. My brother Mike eventually had to get on with his own life. It wasn't fair to keep him tethered to our problems forever. Mike's grandparents took on the reins for a while, in their own quiet way.

Mark went to work like a robot. He told no one. He grieved as much as I did, but silently, and approached the situation academically, gathering information regularly from the internet.

Chapter 17 – Ativan

This medication was prescribed for Mike to control acute anxiety and is frequently used to manage anxious behaviors of psychotic patients in the hospital environment. It was the same medication that was given to Mike on that first evening in the hospital emergency room. It was the "nice shot" that I had promised would help him to "get some sleep," as I tricked him into going to our local hospital for evaluation. We kept the tablets hidden away on the top shelf of our regular medicine cabinet, away from Mike's Abilify, Cogentin, and asthma meds.

Quite frankly, I was afraid of it because I had read on the internet that it was addictive. I had hoped that Mike's Abilify would kick in soon and relieve his symptoms. At bedtime, I gave Mike the smallest dose prescribed, which he found about as helpful as a glass of tap water. Mike reported to his father that this small dose wasn't working as he continued with his restless behaviors at night. Sometimes a little knowledge is dangerous. Mark gave Mike the maximum dose allowed without hesitation, dispensing it as confidently as a teaspoon of cough syrup. It came upon Mike like a club and allowed him to close his eyes for the evening. Upon awakening, Mike said, "It's like I close my eyes for a minute and then it's suddenly morning, but I don't feel as if I ever slept."

Mike's initial diagnosis was "Acute Psychotic Episode." We were told that if his symptoms persisted but lasted less than six months, his diagnosis would then be "Schizophreniform Disorder." If his symptoms persisted after six months, it was indeed schizophrenia, and Mike would have to take medication for the rest of his life. We had kept dialogue with Mike brief about his illness, only describing it as a chemical imbalance in his brain. After about seven weeks, Dr. Kim began to explain the facts to Mike and honestly described to Mike what was happening to him. Dr. Kim rates among the kindest of doctors that I have ever known. He is a kind-faced Korean doctor who somehow chose the lowest paying of all specialties in the medical profession.

Now the cat was out of the bag. Mike's tormenting voices were still there, but the long list of horrendous side effects began to surface before we could make them go away. Mike's realization that he had a devastating disease increased his anxiety. In private, away from his Uncle Mike, he asked both of us to kill him on many occasions. I don't know exactly what he said to his father, but I know what he said to me.

"Mother, do you really want me to live like this? Can't you see that the very best part of me is already dead? I can't feel anything. I have no emotions. I can't even enjoy the beauty of a sunset. I really wanted to be an actor. That's all I ever wanted. It's never been a delusion." With a steady stream of drool running from his mouth, he asked, "How can I do this now, with absolutely no emotions left alive in me? Who will love me or marry me? I'm a modern-day leper. It's like I'm King Midas. You'd give me anything that I wanted and if I touched it, it would all turn into gold, and I couldn't enjoy it anyway. Mom, get me out of this. It would be a mercy killing. I'm already gone from you. Hanging on to me like this is just selfish. Let me go. Help me out of this."

"Mike, if I could, I'd gladly change places with you. Any mother would do this for her child."

"Mom, you're a very strong person, but not strong enough for this."

I looked at him with deep compassion, and thought, *They don't allow animals to suffer like this.* But my response was the same. "Mike, you'll get better. It's just going to take some time."

But on each occasion, I wondered if I wasn't being selfish. Would he ever come back to us? Some people don't. I wondered how long I would be able to watch his suffering. I believed that God allows bad things to happen to good people for His own reasons. Does He want us to learn to be grateful? Or teach us how we must live?

I had always enjoyed the relief I felt from several beers after returning home from work every evening. As the demands for "a way out of this mess" increased, so did my drinking and my own fantasies. I remembered the patient whom I had cared for, years ago at Maple Tree Nursing Home, who heard voices continuously. What kind of a life did she have? I had never been an advocate of abortion, capital punishment, or euthanasia. All of these issues had previously made me more than uncomfortable. It must have been my "motherly response to crying" that even allowed me to ponder such awful ideas.

I thought, *Mike could still drive our boat, given a little direction. We could pack up two pillows and some blankets in the back and drive far out into the lake. We could split a case of beer and that bottle of Ativan that I was so afraid of. It might be enough to do the job.* Mike had been my live baby doll, my little playmate, my grown child and friend whom I respected. Now he was begging for mercy from torment. We could go to sleep, once again holding hands for comfort. It would be mercy. I couldn't take him out and not go with him. I imagined that I would accompany him into the next world, which would be so much better than this one of torture.

Mike had a brain disorder and thus a mental illness; yet I felt like the person who had been driven crazy with grief and rage. Nothing bad happened, because ultimately I feared the pains of hell and my own separation from God. I wanted to be connected with God, and I feared Him. I begged for God's mercy, in both my drunken and sober hours, and attempted to make all kinds of bargains with Him. But it doesn't work that way.

I am convinced that God has His own plans for us, but that He is influenced by the prayers of many. Those prayers came. Later, when I confessed my irrational thoughts during this time to Mark, he was terribly shocked and lamented, "Susie, how could you have ever thought of leaving me alone?"

Chapter 18 – Why I Chose to Tell the Truth to My Customers

First and foremost in my mind, there was absolutely nothing that could ever make me ashamed of my boy. From the day of his birth, he was a gift to us in every sense of the word and brought great joy and fulfillment to our marriage. From the time that he was little, Mike seemed to have an inner wisdom and peace that was far beyond his years. In my mind, he was pretty much a perfect son. This terrible disease could never destroy the profound respect I had for him. I told the truth, therefore, because I felt no shame.

The second and most practical reason that I told the truth was because I needed to stay employed. Mark and I had always been a team as income earners. The realization that we might have to provide for Mike after our own deaths was a compelling factor for me to get back to work as soon as possible. I had tried not to let my customers down, even on the smallest of issues, and they deserved my honesty. They were all my friends. I had to tell them that I might be limping for a while, but that they could still expect the same level of service from me.

The third reason that I told my customers the truth was to educate them. Family is a common denominator in the furniture business and in many of the stores that I called on, their families had been in the business for three generations, just like mine. I found it to be a unique business, with talented people on the retail side who had been groomed to eventually "take over" since they were children. From a young age, they learned how to unload, repair, display, market, and buy products that aren't just functional but are part of the fashion industry. The industry hosts a very large group of multi-talented professionals and has long been called "The Gentleman's Business" for good reason. I explained our circumstances and told them, "If this could happen to Mike, it could happen to anyone." I was amazed at how well-read and self-educated many of them were regarding mental illnesses.

The results of my honesty were incredible. Severe mental illnesses affect one out of five families. Whether they had a personal experience with a loved one or simply knew someone who had a problem, almost all of them offered to pray for us. Many put Mike's name on their own church's prayer list. I realized later, as I tried to do the math, there must have been thousands of people praying for my son.

All of my customers were compassionate and a few openly cried, but one female customer stands out in my mind quite clearly. Despite the fact that she was roughly my own age, something about her reminded me of my mother. My mother was always a straight shooter, very direct. You never had to wonder what she was thinking. My customer's exact words to me were this: "Susie, this is terrible, but you know what doesn't kill you will make you stronger."

Chapter 19 – Prognosis

Dr. Kim began to give Mike more and more information after the seventh week when he could see some clearing in Mike's eyes. They were still bleary and the side effects of his medication were pronounced. It must have been about the ninth week when, out of the blue, Mike asked, "What are my chances?" I was totally shocked as I heard this question. I couldn't believe that he spoke so clearly and definitively. "Dr. Kim, I have taken a lot of courses in mathematics, including calculus along with statistics in college. Do you have a statistical chart or a probability distribution graph that might give me an idea?" I believe that Dr. Kim was as surprised as I. He promptly brought out his medical book and showed Mike his chances for recovery.

"Mike, it's like this," Dr. Kim explained as he pointed to the graph. "Outcomes are broken down into percentages. The disease occurs in 1.1% of the population worldwide."

"25% will have one or two discrete episodes, lasting less than a period of six months. The disease will go away spontaneously."

"25% will have symptoms that last longer than six months and will have to take medication for the rest of their lives. This group can often work full or part-time."

"25% will need a lot of support and can't live totally independently."

"25% will have poor outcomes."

Mark and I had read everything that we could find on schizophrenia. The work by Dr. E. Fuller Torrey, M.D., in his book *Surviving Schizophrenia*, was our best source. We were familiar with these statistics and understood the meaning of the last 25%. 10% would remain symptomatic and institutionalized, and 15% would eventually die, mostly by suicide. I believed then and believe now that this 15% reflects people who are so ill that they can't bear to live with their symptoms, people who can't live with the side-effects of their medications, or people who were once quite gifted and can't live with their loss of functioning.

Mike had leaned forward to view the chart. Now he sat back and looked past Dr. Kim, staring at the wall, convincingly in thought. Then he shook his head in disbelief. "I can't believe that this happened to me," he said, wiping the drool from his mouth. "Dr. Kim, if I take my medication as prescribed and never miss a dose, can I avoid a relapse?"

"No, Mike, I can't guarantee that."

"I don't ever want to go back there, Dr. Kim." Mike asked one more question on this visit. "Would it be fair to say that the longer I go without a relapse, the less my chances are of getting one?"

"That is a fair question, and my answer to that is Yes." Dr. Kim tried to be encouraging. "My patients with schizophrenia do quite well. They go back to college; they work in factories; they get married; and they have children." I could hardly believe what he was saying. I only hoped that Mike would fall into the first 25% and that this terrible nightmare would simply go away. But it didn't.

It would take a full two years and eight months for Mike to get past many of his symptoms and the unbearable side effects of his medications. We were in for the long haul, with absolutely no guarantees. Mike proved to be the bravest man I had ever known, enduring all manner of pain and torture, and then made his second debut as a true hero.

"Do you believe in the power of prayer?" I asked Dr. Kim after a year or two.

"If it works for you, it works for me," he said as he looked at me and smiled with kind eyes. Dr. Kim is such a gentleman. He clearly believed in the power of the correct medication. I didn't bother to tell him that I had prayed to God to inspire him to make the right choices for Mike.

Chapter 20 –The Verdict and the Sentence

After six months, the verdict and the sentence for life came in. Mike continued to have mild hallucinations. Sometimes he saw sparkling small stars in his field of vision. Other times, they were somatic, meaning pertaining to the body and not the mind. He would experience tingling sensations in his nose or waves of pulsating "rushes" going from his forehead down his spine. While these were much milder versions of what he had suffered earlier, they occasionally occurred, showing up at the most unexpected times. Mike's sense of hearing was now extremely acute, and he could hear a train coming long before the rest of us. He worried when he heard house noises, people talking outside our house, or dogs barking. "We heard it too," we'd say as we constantly tried to reassure him. He was afraid to rely on his five senses because they had so convincingly betrayed him in the past. While the verdict and sentence for life was delivered to Mike by Dr. Kim, as parents, Mark and I understood the implications from our reading, both from books and the internet.

- Your child has schizophrenia. This is an incurable disease.
- This disease can be manageable, just like diabetes.
- This disease is still poorly understood by the general population.
- This disease still carries a lot of stigma because people are afraid of schizophrenics.

- The media sensationalizes and exploits any bizarre action or violent crime committed by a person who suffers from schizophrenia.

- Schizophrenics taking medication have the same rate of violent crimes as the general population.

- The media takes little or no responsibility for educating people about brain diseases.

- Our government and schools take little or no responsibility for education about mental illnesses.

- There are genetic factors, as in any other disease, that predispose a person to develop the disease of schizophrenia.

- Viruses, chemicals, and other no-fault environmental factors may trigger the disease.

- The right drugs and the right dose will be a guessing game.

- Most of the medications that help have cruel side effects.

- Healthcare professionals will rely on statistics.

- Statistics will not always accurately predict the outcome for any individual.

- New medications that have proven to be quite helpful have come on the horizon.

- Since older medications are much less expensive, our government may try to force people, who have had their symptoms totally alleviated by the newer drugs, to "try" an older medication to save money. The result of this experiment would be disastrous and would cause a person to "start all over" in the process of their recovery.

- Older medications, while often effective, have even more cruel side effects than the newer medications.

- In spite of the fact that schizophrenia affects 1 out of 100 people, we keep it in the closet.

- National newscasters and politicians "poetically" speak about our "schizophrenic government".

- Comedians use the word "schizophrenic" to make jokes.

- Irresponsible terminology and reporting lead to further ignorance about this disease.

- If mental illnesses were redefined as organic brain diseases and could be openly acknowledged without the threat of loss of opportunity or jobs, we could have more tax-paying citizens.

- Removing the "mystery" of mental illnesses is essential to widespread acceptance that they do indeed exist, and that there is no "blame or shame" attached to them, as with any other medical diseases.

- Our entire healthcare system seems to have decided that people with schizophrenia have poor prognoses and that we shouldn't spend any more money than necessary, while still maintaining that our country is a caring and responsible nation.

Part III – Looking Back
(1959 – 1984)

Chapter 21 – "They" Were Always There

Most of us ignored them. We turned our faces away when we didn't want to embarrass their loving families. The loving families usually tucked their afflicted member discretely away and kept the secret. Excuses were made why Barry lived at home with his mother, even though he was a grown man. The mother who never attended school functions was cared for by her two pre-adolescent daughters in the afternoon so that their father could earn a living. The blatant and babbling schizophrenic teenage girl in our town could not be ignored. She walked the streets talking nonsense and gibberish, but apparently had an active sex life because she had found a boyfriend who also had the same disorder. He simply had a less verbal and quieter version of the disease, following her everywhere and taking her commands. My own cousin developed schizophrenia in her late teens. She was fair of face, an A-plus student, and headed for the convent when the disease struck. To have a nun in the family would have made any Irish Catholic family proud. But it didn't work out that way for ours. The disease seems to strike the nicest of people and does not discriminate between the wealthy and the poor.

My first experience in knowing a person with schizophrenia occurred when I was only five years old. Our charming, small lakefront community had traditional small-town blocks. Mother and Dad had six children in the first six years of their marriage, but I was their caboose, arriving quite unexpectedly seven years after the last. Mother's résumé on parenting was superior with many years of experience to her credit. She understood the importance of giving a child age-appropriate responsibilities along with sensible limitations. I was given the freedom to meet people and explore our small-town block, but not allowed to cross any street without supervision.

Our middle-class neighborhood housed a mature or aging population, so the opportunities to meet other children were somewhat limited. The children who lived on our block did not share the environment I knew and understood. I quickly figured out that our house always smelled like delicious food was cooking while cleaning elements hung in the air. My mother had me sit on her feet as she hung out the upstairs windows, washing them once a month. Once a week, we slept on fresh, crisp sheets that Mom had washed and hung outside to dry or on the multiple clothes lines in our basement. Our home was scrupulously clean, warm, inviting, and smelled good all of the time.

I tried to make friends with the local children but found my experiences to be both disappointing and enlightening at once. Two of the mothers were harsh disciplinarians, spanking for the mildest of infractions at which my mother would have snickered or given a mild scolding. The third mother had four children under the age of five. Their house reeked of garbage and dirty diapers. None of this was for me! At the tender age of five, I gave up seeking children as my friends and discovered that I was surrounded by kind, wonderful, and wise old people. Every day, I visited three houses and was gladly welcomed by unique spirits who loved a happy little girl and tried to educate her about small things. These old people made my life complete on a daily basis and were the first on my mind in the morning as I rolled sleepily out of bed.

I led a charmed life at the age of five. My three older brothers and three older sisters took me along with them everywhere and helped Mom and Dad with household duties and yard tasks. When it was time for my bath at night, my sisters put a squirt of

Ivory dish soap into our claw-footed bath tub, filled it to the brim, and brought my boat and "little people" from my doll-house to soak with me. Once I was a certifiable prune and the water became cold, I yelled that I was ready to get out. My hair was shampooed; then I was towel dried and sent to bed in warm flannel pajamas, never stirring for ten or eleven hours.

Each morning, I rolled out of bed and searched for my mother. I would find her in the basement doing endless loads of wash or in the kitchen preparing for supper. She greeted me with a smile and quickly made me burnt toast with hard, cold butter on top along with an icy cold glass of milk. My face was washed with a warm washcloth, and I was dressed for the weather to "get some fresh air and go out and play." Next she fixed breakfast for Dad and laid out his clothes for the day. I was simply "round three" of her morning duties as she kissed Dad goodbye and I played for a little while with my beloved doll-house. Back to the basement, she descended, and by the time she came up the stairs, I was awake and ready to go on my daily adventures.

"Mom, I'm going to go see my friends."

"Susie, don't stay too long and annoy those old folks, and please, check in with me."

"They like me, Mom," I said, as I skipped out the front door. Every day, I visited three houses on my five-year-old "milk run" as I anticipated the afternoon kindergarten bus arriving sharply at noon.

My first stop was to visit Harold and Mary. Mary was a soft-spoken woman who played the organ in our church and volunteered for every conceivable charity that existed in our parish. Harold was probably my true inspiration to become a future gardener. He loved the earth like it was his mother and explained all of the names and purposes of the vegetables and flowers that he grew on his property. My most vivid memory of Harold was cleaning and cutting up fresh rhubarb, and serving it to me with salt on the side for dipping. "Honey Girl, it's just like celery, only better."

My mouth would pucker as I grinned and agreed.

Harold had a brother, whose name was Wilbur, who lived right around the corner. Wilbur was described as an "old maid" by the neighbors. He owned a duplex that helped with his income after retirement. His aging and blind mother, who was at least ninety years old, spent her days in the upstairs bedroom. She was extremely confused and called for Wilbur all the time. He cared for her tenderly, feeding her, bathing her, and changing her diapers. Wilbur, I realize now, was probably gay and therefore never married. That wouldn't have made a bit of difference to me then, even if I could have understood it, or now, as being gay has never been an issue for me. Wilbur drank beer with salt in it at 10:00 in the morning as he watched his black and white TV that was mounted to the wall of his knotty-pine kitchen.

Over and over and over I heard, "Wilbur, Wilbur, oh Wilbur, please help me!" Wilbur occasionally took me upstairs to talk to "Mom" and told her that a beautiful little girl had come to see her. At the age of five, I watched as he took care of her most basic needs. I saw him change her diapers, kiss her on the forehead, and calm her down with loving words. Sometimes my sister Kathy, who wanted to be a nurse, volunteered to give Wilbur's mother a bed-bath. That was the way of old neighborhoods in America. Random acts of kindness were not rare events, but routine. Wilbur called me "Honey Child" and always had a seven-ounce bottle of 7 Up with potato chips ready for me when I arrived. He patiently listened to my childish dreams and stories each morning. As I left each day, he waved goodbye at his doorstep and asked if I would be back the next day. We both brightened each other's mornings, and I am fairly sure that occasionally he gave me a sip of his beer and described why he liked the salt in it.

My last stop was always to see Mrs. Cowsill. She had the looks and demeanor of an aging angel. Her dress was impeccable – expensive clothes with matching heels every day. Knowing that she was a late riser, I made this house my last visit before Mom expected me home for lunch and preparation for the school bus. In her living room was a baby grand piano which was the joy in her life. On the end table, a beautiful cut-glass dish always held hard candies. I was allowed to hammer out my own made-up melodies on her piano as I ate up as many pieces of hard candy as I could chew and swallow. Occasionally, Mrs. Cowsill's son Barry bounded down the stairs into the foyer.

"What are you doing, Barry?" she would ask.

"I'm going to the basement, Mother." Barry was probably 45 years old, slim and balding. Sometimes she called him into the living room to see me and I told him about the events of my five-year-old's day. He usually looked at me with luminous eyes that seemed almost too bright, smiled, and then quickly got away to his own agenda.

"Why does Barry live with you and what does he do?" I asked Mrs. Cowsill.

"Barry is divorced and retired," she replied. "He's here to look after me, dear."

"What does Barry do in the basement?"

"Dear, his hobbies are down there."

"Does Barry drive a car?" I asked this apparently odd question because I knew that she walked and pulled a foldable cart along with her to do her shopping.

"Only at night," she replied. She was probably the most patient soul I had ever met. One day, when I came to visit, she looked stern, which was highly unusual.

"Dear, if you come here to visit me and I don't answer the door, do not go inside the house. Do you understand me?"

"Yes," I said. That day came, and I could see that something wasn't right. Barry answered the door with eyes that looked angry and suspicious. He told me that his mother wasn't home.

"It's nice to see you, Mr. Cowsill," I replied. "Please tell your mother that I called." I skipped quickly down the nine steps that led to the front porch of their two-story brick house and turned to wave goodbye, but the door was already shut. I knew somehow that I had been in a dangerous situation and had escaped. So Barry was the first person I met that had this dreadful disease. I was only five years old. My instincts were good at five.

Chapter 22 – My Experiences as a Hospital Nurse

In 1976, I graduated from a well-recognized school of practical nursing. I was not a "born nurse" but a "made nurse." My large Irish Catholic family involved a range of 21 years between the first and the last born. It is the tradition among "old school Irish" to make a place for their boys and to hope that their girls will marry well. My father, the patriarch in our family furniture business, brought his sons, one by one, to "market" and found placements for them as manufacturer's reps in the furniture industry. Appropriate jobs for women at the time were nurses, teachers, hairdressers, and secretaries, and I was supposed to choose from these categories. I don't believe that any of my sisters or I held a grudge. It was simply the way that it was "supposed to be" in our culture. I recall saying to my father, "Dad, I can carry a bag as well as the rest of the boys."

"Suzer (his pet name for me), this is not a business for women." Case closed. He might have been quite surprised if he could have later looked down from heaven to see the course that my life would eventually take. Roughly ten years of nursing caused rapid "burn-out" and led me into a decade of medical sales. Then followed another decade in the furniture business; not only did I carry the same bag as my brothers, but worked his territory as I called on the children of his former dealers. But the result of this conversation was that I obeyed Dad, tried to make him proud of me, and entered a nursing school.

It was a 12-month program of study, which I felt was comprehensive and intense on the "body systems level." In contrast to a registered nurse program, we did not delve deeply into the cellular or chemical aspects of organ functions. Clinical rotations involved hands-on nursing experiences on medical, orthopedic, pediatric, and OB floors along with experience in surgery and Recovery Room. One-day visits were provided to a nursing home, a facility for the mentally and physically handicapped, a hospital emergency room, and a psychiatric ward. These brief rotations were nothing more than exposure to additional opportunities for employment.

During our one-day rotation to a psychiatric unit, we were only allowed to observe. We were not allowed to initiate any conversation but advised to write down what patients said to us. There was no "adding to or subtracting from" any conversation with a patient. Looking back, I realize that this small unit housed patients who suffered from severe neuroses and that there was not a single psychotic patient to observe. The patients with severe mental illnesses were shipped to a hospital an hour away, which was better equipped to handle such matters.

Our pre-clinical lessons and readings were far more informative. We read and learned about all the major mental illnesses with interest and compassion. We studied Sigmund Freud, who was described in 1976 as "The Father of Psychiatry", and read about his concept of "The Ego, Super-Ego, and Id." I memorized what was necessary to pass the test, and tried over and over to digest what he had proposed but couldn't believe his teachings. I don't know why I thought this at the tender age of 22, but my gut instincts were that his teaching were all creative thinking and simply rubbish.

How could he presume to understand what was going on in the human mind? How could he understand the functions of the human brain? How did he come up with such fantastic ideas, and how was he able to get other doctors to embrace them?

While I respect Freud's endeavor to explain diseases of the mind, there were no scientific tools available to substantiate his beliefs. Today we know that there are indeed documentable

changes in the brains of people suffering from both schizophrenia and Alzheimer's disease, and that they are in fact
medical diseases. Some of these changes can be observed on
MRIs (magnetic radiographic images) and sadly, others are seen
on autopsy.

Time went on and I graduated near the top of my class. My
state board scores were even better. I had always been good at
taking tests. This score made me readily employable, and
immediately I was hired for first shift on the floor of my choice,
which was an orthopedic floor. I chose this specialty first,
because of my love for old people. The majority of the patients
that we admitted were elderly, suffered from a fracture, had
surgery, recovered, and went home. These glorious old souls
were grateful for the comfort and kindness of "old school"
bedside nursing care, conversation, and had tons of wonderful
stories to tell. It was a great pleasure to relieve their pain, help
them bathe, and get them moving in the right direction to return
to their own homes. I was happily in the company of "old
people" once again.

The second reason I had chosen this specialty was because
patients rarely died. Even the young people that were admitted to
our floor after a horrific car crash or motorcycle accident would
live. They had already survived the accident, emergency room
care, and surgery before we ever saw them. It was then our job
to keep them on the mend, and sometimes it would take months
before we could discharge them and happily wave goodbye.

Sometimes we got the overflow of patients from medical
floors. They suffered from gall bladder problems, diabetes,
burns, blood clots, stomach ulcers, kidney and chronic heart
problems, along with every imaginable medical disease. Some
had cancer. I had chosen orthopedics as my specialty for good
reason. I knew that I was too soft to cope with the calamities of
the very young or the terminally ill. I simply wanted to provide
care and healing to patients I felt comfortable with, to the best of

my ability. I believed that nursing was a "mothering art" and wanted to practice my art with the elderly. I was absolutely void of any desire to become high-tech or to handle catastrophe on a daily basis.

Occasionally we admitted a patient with a primary diagnosis of schizophrenia, who also had some other ailment, and should have gone to a medical floor. None of them was dangerous in any sense of the word. They were all extremely laid-back and quiet. These patients seldom laughed, but I did my very best to be jovial and tried to get a good smile. I remember well their flaccid faces and stiff fingers. Those were in the days that "smoking rooms" were still available in hospitals. These schizophrenic patients smoked continuously and drank as much coffee as you could bring to them. I was always a clown as I delivered my nursing care and attempted to provide some humor as they recovered from their current ailment. I felt that I was a huge success when I achieved a sincere chuckle.

At the time, all that I knew about schizophrenia was that it was known as "The Young Person's Disease." I knew these patients developed dementia and mental deterioration, usually in their early twenties, at the prime of their lives, and that the disease left them debilitated forever. It was unclear to me whether it was the disease itself or the medications that made people with schizophrenia lack the energy or the initiative to work and remain independent. I simply knew that it was true. I had never heard of a good outcome for schizophrenia and believed that everyone who suffered from the disease either lived with loving family members or in institutions. If there were any survivors of this dreadful disease, they certainly didn't announce themselves.

Stigma was rampant and the ideology about what actually caused a "weak mind" was filled with blame and shame, especially for the schizophrenic's mother. Fear was another factor that would have suppressed survivors from disclosing their disease. The general population believed that schizophrenics were always dangerous and aggressive. I witnessed none of these behaviors. Thorazine, a drug that was used as a medication before surgery, was accidentally discovered to be effective in controlling the positive symptoms such as delusions and hallucinations. Other first-generation antipsychotics followed, and while they controlled the confused symptoms, they had devastating side effects. In my young mind, this was a sad and tragic disease with few alternatives.

Less than two years passed. My father was diagnosed with lung cancer along with metastatic brain cancer. Dad went through a horrific surgery along with radiation therapy and suffered terrible side effects, but still maintained the posture of a positive man. All eight of us visited him as often as possible and used our Irish background of story-telling to keep him amused and laughing. Dad lasted exactly six months after his diagnosis.

On the evening that Dad died in his own bed, his wife and three of "his girls" – my sisters, Kathy and Nan, and I – were by his side. On this occasion, only females were in attendance. I recall my mother holding his hand and saying, "Joe, let go. Don't struggle so hard." Shortly after, Dad spoke for the very last time.

"Hi Ma!" he said, as if he was simply returning home from school. Maybe that's all that this life is – just school.

They say that women are the stronger of the two sexes, and I believe this to be true. My mother, my two sisters, and I had a good cry of relief that Dad was finally out of his misery. A lion-hearted man had left us that evening. The task of "guiding a soul out" has always been "women's work." We are made for this tough assignment because we understand how difficult it is to "guide a new soul in."

Still, our jobs were not yet done. Kathy and I tenderly bathed Dad's dead body with Sweetheart soap before we called the funeral home. I closed his eyes, which had somehow remained slightly open after his death. Nan comforted Mother and distracted her in the kitchen as Kathy and I performed routine post-mortem care. I remember that tender night. Dad's body was sent to the mortuary with dignity and smelling clean. We never covered his face with a sheet or allowed his death to become a macabre event.

Looking at my father's remains caused me to remember him as a person. As strong and unrelenting as he was in his work ethic, Dad had also been quite a character and one hilarious guy. Our street, one of the oldest in town, was paved with red bricks, and most of the houses that lined it, turn-of-the-century vintage. Ours was located almost directly across from "O'Malley Funeral Home." For years, Dad came home on Friday afternoon from his weekly travels as a furniture rep.

"Katy, bring me a highball. I'm tired!" He sat on our tall, pillared porch, put his feet up and enjoyed the weather when it was fair. Usually Dennis O'Malley was grooming his front lawn when Dad called him over for a drink and some town gossip. Dennis was always willing to comply when he could, but sometimes he was on his way out, in his hearse, probably to pick up a corpse. On these occasions, Dad would call out to him from his comfortable chair, "Dennis, I'm not ready yet! When I'm ready, I'll walk across the street, raise my hands into the air, and turn myself in!" Dennis always laughed. But on the night that we called his funeral home to pick up Dad's body, he didn't come. This death was "too close to home" in many ways. Instead, he sent the younger men.

After the removal of Dad's body, Kathy and Nan changed the sheets so that Mother could sleep in the bed she had shared with her husband of many years. I understood as I watched my older sisters quickly put the room in order that this was more of a quiet and symbolic event than a practical one. They were gently telling Mom, "This is where you belong." That night, Mom slept alone for the first time in a long time.

When my father died, my three older brothers were at the International Furniture Market. Dad had told them in advance, "Go! Do your job. I don't want all of you sitting around like a bunch of ghouls waiting for me to die. You'll find out when you need to know." My brothers were all gallant and strong men, but none of them were capable of watching Dad hemorrhage and bleed out to his death. It fell upon me to call "the boys" and after numerous attempts to reach them by telephone, I finally reached Jim and told him that Dad had died around 7:30. I asked him to please tell Mike and Joe, and to come home as soon as they possibly could to help Mom plan the funeral.

My mother, my sisters, and I sat around the kitchen table that night into the wee hours, telling funny and heart-warming stories about Dad. We slept that night from exhaustion and relief, knowing full well that Mother wanted "her boys" at home to take charge and plan the funeral. That was the way of our culture. She would feel safe in their decisions. Then the waiting began, as each of our siblings arrived separately. We'd all be together again. The difference was that Dad would not be there praising us, yelling at us, and shouting commands which we mirthfully laughed at but lovingly obeyed.

The Irish wake for Dad would happen with my brothers and male cousins competing for the best jokes as we drank beer and wiped away the tears. We would all cry and laugh and tell hilarious stories about the man we loved, who happened to be our father. Most importantly, we'd all be together. That was all that Mom and Dad had ever wanted. They never wanted us to be separated for any reason.

I remembered a story my mother had told me when I was a teenager. Mom and Dad had taken on a huge debt to open their furniture store. They had sold almost everything that they owned to accomplish this task. They also changed their wills. In the case of both their deaths, all of us children were to be kept together. Our parents understood that there were many well-meaning relatives who might "step up" for one child, but no one could take on seven. So they picked out an orphanage where we could all be kept together. That is how strongly they felt about the bond that they wanted to survive in their family.

We followed a plow truck to the cemetery and buried our father in the midst of a blizzard. The winter of 1978 was as vicious as I can remember of any winter. The grave-side service was short because even the priest decided that the weather was extreme.

After my father's long and painful death, I needed a change. I no longer had any desire to take care of cancer patients overflowing onto my orthopedic floor. I had chosen orthopedics for a sound reason. I knew what I was doing right from the start. I had never wanted to take care of babies, children, or young people with no chance of survival. I simply wasn't up to that task and knew it. If a ninety-year-old person happened to die, I could deal with it. *Didn't that person have the opportunity to have a full life?*

I was good at making people comfortable. I wasn't good at dealing with tragedy that involved young people who never had the chance for happiness or a full life. I knew that I was a complete and total coward in this area of nursing, and I had successfully avoided it.

I applied for a position in the hospital, which involved working in an orthopedic clinic, and I was accepted. My responsibilities also included setting up all of the "skin traction" in the entire hospital, and I was allowed to work quietly and independently. It seemed to be "the perfect job." But there's always a "rub" in any perfect position. I also had to help out in the emergency room. Off I went "from the frying pan into the fire."

I don't know what I could have been thinking when I eagerly pursued this position. I wasn't cut out to be a trauma nurse! Certainly I could help with the usual sore throats, earaches, and lacerations that presented themselves at our door. No big deal. Most of the major accidents came in on the 3 to 11 shift or on the 11 to 7 shift, but I saw my share, and this job wasn't for me. Maybe the hospital environment wasn't my calling. I didn't want to feel like a "quitter", so I stuck with this job for a year. By then, I had seen enough and put in my resignation.

It was during my last two weeks that a certain young man presented himself in the waiting area of the emergency room. He couldn't have been more than 25 years old. His head was turned up to the right and his eyes were rolled back in his head, just like a doll. He spoke through clenched teeth, everything from his neck up distorted because of muscle contractions. "I want to see the doctor," he said with contortion of all the muscles that involved his face and neck. Horrified, I asked our emergency room doctor to please come out and look at the young man. The physician took one look and told the admitting secretary to forget the paperwork for now. He took the young man by the arm and brought him to a gurney.

"Nurse, now! Cogentin 2 mg, IM stat, and I mean now!" The drug was administered by injection within a minute and within ten minutes, the ghoulish distortion dissipated. I had never seen anything up to this date so frightening, even with all the blood and guts, which now had become second-nature to this troubling job. Our ER doctor quietly spoke to the young man, "You must speak to your psychiatrist about your medication." Dr. Johnson walked away, put his head down and quietly wiped away a tear. I heard him say to himself, under his breath, "Poor guy."

Dr. Johnson was a man of great compassion, and I had only seen him cry openly and unashamedly on one other, very recent occasion. It was the day that I had decided to rectify the bad decision that I had made, taking a position for which I was so completely unsuited. At 7:30 that morning, I had closed the eyes of a teenager who had been in a car accident. His injuries were internal and no matter how much blood Dr. Johnson poured into him, more came out. Our beloved doctor had worked on him all night.

But now I had seen an "acute dystonic reaction" to an antipsychotic medication. I was more terrified by this sight than I had been by other "blood and guts" suffering and sudden death situations. I witnessed first-hand the consequences a schizophrenic faces, not just from the disease but also from the medication.

It had only been a few weeks before this event that I was approached by Sally, a registered nurse who had worked with me on St. Anthony's, my old orthopedic floor. She was most likely in her late thirties, and was slightly chubby, very blonde, and freckly. I remembered that she had always been extraordinarily kind. Sally had been a team player, always on the sidelines, and had never become involved in politics that occurs on hospital wards.

"Susie, rumor has it that you're not very happy in the ER. You love old people, and you are very good with them. You should get a job in a nursing home. You'd really enjoy it and have a lot of fun as a charge nurse. You'd have a lot of responsibility, and you're capable of more responsibility."

"Sally, how did you know that I was unhappy?"

"It's written all over your face."

Angels always come in the most peculiar forms. I took Sally's advice and went on to some of the happiest years of my entire life. I never saw Sally again, but her face is written in my heart.

Chapter 23 – Five Years at Maple Tree Nursing Home

I was lovingly welcomed aboard by Molly Below, the Director of Nursing at Maple Tree Nursing Home. Molly was one of the kindest and most easy-going nurses that I have met. Almost nothing ruffled her feathers. Her kind spirit, good nature, and wholesomeness were married with years of practical decisions involving nursing, mothering, and farming. She was probably about fifty at the time, slightly robust in frame, with dark brown hair, beautiful skin, and a smiling face. Molly was truly "salt of the earth" in every sense of the word and proved to be the best of bosses and also a very good friend.

My five years at Maple Tree brought along with me some profound life experiences and changes. Molly kept me employed and made accommodations in my schedule as I went through a divorce early on, then later a remarriage, a miscarriage, and the birth of my only child. I believe that it would also be fair to say that I was a responsible nurse and that she respected my work ethic, managing skills, and desire to give our residents the best possible care.

Maple Tree was a 100-bed facility, with 50 beds on the east wing, which housed the more ambulatory residents who simply needed a whole lot of assistance. The west wing was for our more acutely ill residents who were for the most part bed or chair-ridden. Through the years, I worked on both wings with shifts on 7-3 and 3-11.

The nurses at Maple Tree willingly accepted me. The nursing assistants were my hardest nuts to crack. They were small-town and "farm-fed" strong girls and women, and I had to prove myself to them! Most of them had been working in the facility since its inception. I was new and, for a while, I was challenged by them. They were testing me. It didn't take me too long to figure out that after my morning or afternoon nurse's report, I should report to them! At the end of the shift, I asked for their advice. "What do you think that we should do to help Mrs. Jones?" It was so easy! I had empowered them, and they returned the favor. They ultimately understood that I was responsible for what happened during my watch, but that I relied on their good sense and wisdom. We all became good friends and a strong working team.

The 7-3 shift was more of a challenge than 3-11. Day shift included the two major meals of the day, two important medication passes, and often doctors' rounds. Transports to optometrists, dentists, and other specialists had to be arranged. Family members of our residents often took them out for a few hours or days. All the paperwork had to be in order along with dispensing necessary medications for the period of time they would be gone. Enjoyable but time-consuming activities were provided daily by our activity department. Pharmacists could show up at any time and needed attention. There were tube-feedings, treatments, and dressing changes. What I have outlined involves a "good day."

I preferred working 3-11, which was much more relaxed as our residents were winding down from a busy day. The supper meal and a bedtime snack were much easier. Few doctors came, and fewer activities were scheduled. Aside from routine skilled nursing duties which remained the same, the only additional responsibility was the notorious "BM List." Patients who had not "gone" in the last three days were given a laxative or suppository. This was the best shift to visit with our folks, listen to their stories, and let them know that we loved them. I enjoyed pushing my medication cart on the evening med pass, after the nursing assistants had delivered bedtime snacks. I got to give not only pills but also a delicious "home-baked" tasting cookie and juice.

It had been considered unprofessional in the hospital to sit down on a chair in a patient's room. To sit on a patient's bed was taboo! But at Maple Tree, I made my own rules about what was appropriate, depending on the resident. I did sit on the side of their bed sometimes and offered the snack first, pills later. I always asked: "How are you feeling?", "How did your day go?", "Do you need anything?" I wanted to be in a position of eye contact and not above the residents. This quiet time in the evening gave me more information about any particular resident than any other clue during the day.

Many of the old ladies hugged me and kissed me on the cheek. I often kissed some of the ladies and gents on the forehead or held their hand after their meds and "tucked them in." Some of them had a "blue" day. They missed their spouses, their homes, their children or more sadly, their deceased children. They missed their independence and friends, and sometimes cried because they were "the last ones." They had outlived all of the people that they loved. I think it was enough sometimes to simply say, "I know." Other times, it was better to say, "You are having a bad day. Tomorrow will be better."

I have described normal and "good" days on both shifts. A "bad" day was when someone fell down and had to be transported to the hospital for stitches or a broken hip, had a stroke or heart attack, vomited blood, became unconscious for unknown reasons, or died unexpectedly. This is truly an abbreviated list of potential calamities.

A really "bad" month was when one resident got an upper respiratory infection, a gastrointestinal infection, or the actual flu. When one was infected, they all became infected and so did the staff. Our nurses poured medications into our residents, watched their vital signs, and shipped them off to the hospital when necessary. Our nursing assistants cleaned them up relentlessly, poured fluids into them, and came to work even when they were sick right beside them. We had our own little community within our local community, and took care of "our own" to the best of our abilities and weathered the storms that came. During these bouts of community infections, we lost a few of our beloved old people who didn't have the physical stamina to fight off the infections.

The worst epidemic came when I was pregnant with Mike, in my sixth month. We poured liquid Tylenol for fevers and cough syrups that were expectorants into everyone. Those dignified old people were suddenly weakened, pleading children. I came to work, never missed a day, and coughed right along with everyone else. I didn't take any medication because I was afraid that it might hurt my developing baby. My obstetrician did not prescribe an antibiotic because I was able to cough up mucus and keep my airways open. However, I had been really sick for a solid month. I believed at the time, that through my years of nursing, my immune system was pretty well developed. I believed that I could rely on my baby's placenta to filter out the rest of infectious agents.

It would be a huge mistake to describe our community as simply taking care of the basic needs of old people. These "old people" weren't dead yet! Our staff knew all about their lives, and the residents knew all about ours. They took pleasure in our weddings and babies and felt compassion for our tragedies. Truly, we were all something of an extended family.

Old people know everything! They all knew when I got divorced. They all knew when I remarried and when I suffered a miscarriage. They all relished as my abdominal girth increased with each month of my pregnancy with my baby who would become "Mike." I worked until almost the bitter end and could barely waddle down the corridors. Before my pregnancy, I weighed 104 pounds and was 5'1" tall. By the time of my delivery, I weighed in at a whopping 154 pounds. I looked like a balloon that floated in and out of doorways, leaning backwards to keep my balance.

Mike was a very active baby in the womb. When I was walking, he would remain comforted and "rocked." At the very moment I sat down to rest, Mike was like a "kick boxer." So the fun of it was that I would enjoy asking our residents if they would like to feel my belly.

"My baby is really bouncing around right now. Want to see?" No one refused, even the old men. They put their hands on my belly and grinned. Life is renewed in the most ordinary ways! They felt the drums beating, laughed out loud, and asked what I would name my baby. I asked them all for suggestions and this opened up further dialogue.

"I like you so much that I would like to sit on your lap," I would say jestingly to some of my favorites as they sat in the lounge watching television.

"No, no, you are way too fat!" they cried out amidst their hilarious laughter.

So who were these glorious old souls and why were they in this institution? Most of them were simply old. Along with "simply old" came the ailments of the old – dementia, along with other major organ diseases. Everyone had arthritis. Almost no one could see or hear well. Their body organs were worn out and didn't function as well as they used to. Some had suffered from strokes or heart problems. They were with us because either their children were still working and couldn't take care of them, or their children didn't want the responsibility. Some had no children. All of these problems were sad, and it was our job to "make a life" for them. In spite of these facts, the "merely old" residents were not the saddest residents of all.

I was surprised when I first hired on that no less than 10 to 15% of our residents had a primary diagnosis of schizophrenia. Molly, the Director of Nursing, had told me early on that tons of patients had recently been released from mental institutions because they were no longer deemed harmful or dangerous in any way. Nursing homes had absorbed many of these patients who had been institutionalized for years. I remember all of their faces and their names. None of them was ever dangerous in any way. All of them were on first-generation antipsychotics including Thorazine, Stellazine, Haldol, and Mellaril, and others. Almost all of them had some degree of "Tardive dyskinesia." Tardive dyskinesia is a profound side effect of antipsychotic drugs that involves involuntary muscular movements, usually confined to the face, with chewing, sucking, and blowing or tongue rolling actions of the mouth. Sometimes it is even more severe and involves the entire body with relentless and continuous writhing or involuntary movements. Some residents were much worse than others.

On the east wing, we had "Henry" who was on Stellazine. His face was so flaccid that we couldn't keep his eyes lubricated because his lower lids hung down like a bloodhound's. His knees bounced relentlessly when he was seated. He was not a particularly pleasant man. But who would be if life had been robbed at twenty years of age, with the last fifty spent in an institution? Henry shuffled when he walked, drooled constantly, and never seemed able to connect with his care-givers. On the west wing, we had a resident named "Elsie". She was also about seventy years old. Even at this age, I could tell that in her youth, she had been quite beautiful. Her skin was absolutely flawless. She could have been the Bo Derek of her time, given the chance. Instead, she hallucinated continuously, writhing non-stop from full-body Tardive dyskinesia. The only time this writhing stopped was when she slept. Her "voices" were with her at all waking times, and she answered them constantly. Elsie conversed with her voices all day long. All of the rest of our schizophrenic population rested in their beds for most of the day, smoked heavily, and drank copious amounts of coffee.

It wasn't until many years later that I realized that their "need" for caffeine and nicotine was more than a superficial weakness. They relied on these chemicals that stimulated their brains and somehow caused better functioning. They roused for meals, card games, and weekly Mass. They understood "The Body of Christ." I always found this completely touching that they found such comfort in The Eucharist. Most of them walked with a shuffling gait, and had poor posture and stiff fingers. It was a great achievement to get any of them to smile when you tried to be light. In spite of their tragic lives, they were also a valuable part of our small community, and we tried our best to make them feel loved. Looking back, their days at Maple Tree Nursing Home were most likely the best days of their lives, since they became ill in their youth. The mental institutions in those earlier days were probably the closest thing to Hell that could be experienced on this earth.

Once again, Molly rescued me. "Susie, I'm not sure that you can push that heavy medication cart around any longer. You're getting too big with your pregnancy. I have some extra hours in my budget to spend. What do you think that you could do to contribute and to help us?" I understood immediately that Molly knew that I had to stay employed and that my husband and I needed the money. What a benevolent spirit she was!

"Molly, the nursing assistants do a really great job keeping our residents clean and free of problems. The only thing I believe we are lacking is the care of our residents' fingernails. I could soak their hands, trim all of their fingernails, and file and paint our lady residents' fingernails."

"That's a really great idea," Molly replied. "I'll let our newly-hired girl take over as charge nurse. You can help her along too." Molly's plan was to get my replacement oriented with a token amount of help from me and let me leave, after five years of service, with dignity. After our baby was born, we planned to move closer to the city where Mark had signed a contract as a math teacher.

My belly had grown so huge that I had to spread my knees to give it room as I groomed the fingernails of our residents. It was difficult to get close to them. I had completed manicures for at least ten ladies, and then concentrated on the men. Henry was next. I soaked his hands in warm soapy water for fifteen minutes. His fingernails were long and terribly discolored by the stain of tobacco from cigarettes. After the soaking, I brought out the clippers and started chopping away. Henry was complacent until I cut too close and he felt a pinch. No blood was drawn, or I would have filled out an "incident report." Henry, who had always been completely compliant, raised his fist to me and appeared ready to deliver.

"Please Henry, don't hurt the baby," I implored.

Henry lowered his fisted hand and offered it to me in a relaxed position to continue. In spite of Henry's diagnosis, I still felt that he was not a danger. Now, he was simply a confused old man.

In my wildest imagination, I could not have conceived on that day that the child I was carrying would eventually develop the same disease as Henry. The very thought of it would have been too painful to endure as I hopefully awaited the birth of our baby. I had never seen or heard of a person who had recovered from this terrible disease. This was in the year 1984.

Part IV – Michael's Recovery

Chapter 24 – Lois

Lois is more than my cleaning lady. She is a best friend in time of need. When my mother died out-of-state, her body was returned to her place of birth, which was our home town. All my siblings gathered at our home to celebrate Mom's life and lay her body to rest next to our father's in a small rural cemetery. Lois immediately recognized my urgent need and, even though she had worked for another client that day, cleaned my entire house and changed all of the beds. She tried to refuse payment but was not allowed that concession. On the day of Mother's wake, Lois brought tons of food and slipped quietly away, not allowing us the opportunity to express our gratitude. In short, Lois is an angel walking this earth without wings.

Lois is also a woman whose intelligence cannot be dismissed. While I did not openly announce to her what had happened to Mike, she knew. She came on time, as usual, every other Wednesday, and took care of all of our heavy cleaning needs. Lois is quite unique in that whatever you bargained for in the way of household help, she always gave more. She would see a need and simply fulfill it.

Upon seeing Mike on her first visit, after his discharge from the hospital, she immediately asked, "Mike had a nervous breakdown, didn't he?"

"Yes, Lois, he did."

Lois came from a very large family and openly announced, "The same thing happened to one of my brothers. He's still not right. He talks to himself."

"How old is he, Lois?"

"He's fifty-five and lives with one of my sisters down south. She looks after him." She was very sad for us.

As time went on and Mike realized what had happened to him, his innate intelligence increased his anxieties. "Mom, you're not going to live forever. I don't want to die in an institution."

"You won't, Mike. We'll make sure of that. You're going to get better, but it'll take some time." Our reassurances continued whether we were absolutely certain or not. We investigated long-term plans for Mike after our deaths and hoped that we would never have to follow through.

Mike began to rally near the end of October. "Mike looks just like himself," Lois remarked. The miracle we were waiting for was occurring: Mike was coming back to this world. My siblings gently urged me to release our brother Mike from his brotherly-motherly responsibilities.

"Let him go now, Susie. Mike's getting better."

My brother Mike came for another two weeks. Then I knew that I had to let him go and live his own life. He had saved us from financial ruin and worry about Mike's daily care and survival. He had literally held my hand as I cried loudly and uncontrollably, and drank myself into peaceful oblivion. He was the only one who understood why. It had been that horrible to watch.

On the next Wednesday that Lois came to clean, I said to her, "Lois, I'm still so afraid. I have to keep working, and it's hard for me to leave Mike alone. At the present time, I'm making a lot of money. Would you consider working full-time for me and simply taking care of Mike and my house? I would pay you anything you asked."

"Why don't you wait and see what happens?" Lois said as she wisely gave me a hug. Somehow, she was confident that things would turn out all right. I was still worried about the possibility that Mike would gas himself in the garage. Only I knew that he had been thinking about this solution.

Chapter 25 – Could it Happen to You?

One day ran together with the next. Then weeks flowed by like a river as the veil slowly lifted from Mike's mind. Improvement couldn't be measured by either a day or a week; but as time marched on, we understood that Mike was getting better. It was a much better measuring stick to grade his return to health in 90-day intervals.

Routine household responsibilities of our Monday through Friday work-week had been assumed for months exclusively by my brother Michael. Still, the weekends held unavoidable duties. Mark and I stood watchful guard over our son, spelling each other for periods of time so that mundane tasks could be accomplished. Mark had been a devoted husband, companion, and father for many years. Together we had been through many troubled times and had somehow made things work out, but this obstacle seemed insurmountable to us.

Banking, mailing, dry cleaning, oil changes for our cars, grocery shopping, haircuts, and paying bills had always been the demands of our weekends. Some things never change even when there is a major tragedy or crisis going on. In addition to paying the bills online, doing laundry, and cooking meals, Mark devoted most of his waking hours searching the internet for websites that could offer us information and advice. Through a NAMI (National Alliance on Mental Illness) website, Mark found a list of highly recommended books. Mark ordered twelve of them, and later we both read them all, cover to cover. Mark also found a NAMI contact locally, which later led us to get involved in a support group and meet some of the finest people in the world.

In his academic way, Mark got our family on the road to recovery. On Saturdays, he released me to accomplish some of the domestic tasks that kept the ball rolling in our house.

For many Saturdays, the routine was exactly the same. I kissed Mike goodbye and told him that I would be gone for a couple of hours to run errands. "Dad is here to look after you," I said as Mike looked at me through bleary eyes.

Drooling, Mike asked, "Mom, do you think I'm ready to go back to my modeling and acting school?"

"No, not yet, Mike. I think that we should wait a little while longer. I'll tell you when I think you're ready. OK?"

"OK, Mom." Each time, I left with bile in my throat.

The worst times for me were my trips to WalMart or the grocery store. I remembered all the trips I had taken with Mike when he was little, accomplishing the exact same tasks. Each Saturday held the excitement of some little toy that Mike wanted at our local Hills department store. He had been allowed to pick out one small trinket as we waited to get his hair cut and purchased other necessities. Then we proceeded to Kroger's, where the key treasure was a box of animal crackers in a festive carton on a string. The grand finale had been a couple of rides on the bouncing electrical "horsey" on our way out the door. The promise of one ride made Mike behave throughout the ordeal of grocery shopping for the week. Two or three rides were even better when I successfully searched the bottom of my purse for additional loose quarters. What an adventure it had been, and what fun we had during those days doing such ordinary things!

But now I looked at the world through different eyes. Sadly, I watched other parents with their infants, babies, and children. I heard how the parents spoke kindly to their young ones and realized that this was their own Saturday adventure. They were no different than we were years ago. I listened to their sweet dialogues and envied my own past.

I have always enjoyed other people's children from a distance. In the checkout lines, it was always the same. I couldn't help myself as I made eye contact with the babies and children who were worn out from their family's shopping expedition. I smiled and curved my fingers down and waved at them waiting. They all liked my quiet attention and smiled, waved back, and asked for more smiles and waves as they waited patiently in the seat of their shopping cart. I always complied, but then thought about their parents, hard-working people trying to do the right thing for their kid. *I hope it turns out OK for you*, I thought. Secretly, I wished them well as I considered the statistics: one out of one hundred. Then, as I looked at their baby, I wondered: "Could it happen to you?"

Chapter 26 – The World's Greatest Actor

November came and all of Mike's blatant "positive symptoms", meaning delusions and bizarre hallucinations, were gone. And yet a whole new set of conditions would confront us. Mike was right. *It is the disease that keeps on giving.*

We were now facing all of the "negative symptoms" such as blunted or flat emotions, "avolition", or a lack of motivation, and a small degree of "alogia", or poverty of speech. Sometimes Mike was slow to respond to a question, and his spontaneity was diminished. Far and away, the worst of his negative symptoms was "anhedonia," which means he was completely unable to experience pleasure. In my mind, pleasure meant joy.

With all that had happened to Mike, anxiety was a major issue. Trauma from his acute psychotic experience and confirmation of his illness, along with the vicious side effects of his medications, would have made any young man anxious. Mike understood that he had a pronounced loss of functioning, but his worst fear was whether the disease would come back to fully manifest. Mike spent many hours each day lying quietly in his bed, allowing his brain injury to heal and escaping mental stimulation. "Gating", that is, filtering out background noises, remained a continuous problem in his attention abilities. In a loud open room such as a restaurant, Mike couldn't "hear" what we were saying, as all of the sounds ran together and could not be separated.

Part of my prayers had been answered. The voices were gone. Each day, I looked on my boy with new pity as I saw the "ghost of Michael" who now walked among us. One set of tortures had been replaced by another. I often wondered: *This is what has been left to us?*

In spite of all of his residual "negative" symptoms, one day in late November, Mike announced that he thought he was ready to return to modeling and acting school.

"Michael, I want you to believe that you can still try to be anything that you want to be."

I called Mrs. Augustine. After all, we had paid for Mike's lessons in advance. "Mrs. Augustine, can Mike return to his lessons?"

"Are you sure that he's ready, Susie?"

"He's much better now, Mrs. Augustine," I replied with complete conviction. Internally, I felt nothing less than panic.

"Good. We start a new group of male modeling students on December 8th. We'll look forward to coaching and representing Mike. He has a good look."

For the next eight weeks, excluding Christmas break, I drove Mike into the city for one-hour lessons each Tuesday night at 7 o'clock. The lessons were not terribly challenging and might best be described as "finishing school" for young men. Manners, dressing correctly, walking on a cat-walk, and other demands of male models were discussed. Mike was able to complete the eight-week regimen without any problems. The class involved a small group of young men, perhaps a dozen. The interaction was for the most part quiet. I proudly snapped pictures of Mike at his "graduation ceremony," as he walked the cat-walk in three different outfits and posed for the audience of proud, paying parents. Far and away, he was the best looking young man in his group.

Then for six months, Mike attended acting lessons on Saturdays, from noon until 3:00 PM. Weekly, I dropped him off with all of his materials and made sales calls in the city and its suburbs. Mark and I had read that while schizophrenia is a medical disease and is not caused by stress, stressful circumstances can exacerbate (aggravate or increase) symptoms and trigger a relapse. I drove away, each time trembling and praying that nothing would go "wrong". Would he get confused? Would he be able to respond spontaneously? I knew he couldn't sometimes. Would they think that he was shy, or would they figure it out? Clearly we had to keep the disease a secret or Mike would have absolutely no chance to at least try to achieve his dream. Whether his dream was realized or not was inconsequential to me. I had long ago told him that his chance at becoming an actor was about one in a million. What I cared about now was his desire to try.

"Michael, just because you got this terrible disease, you can't give up. Your chances are still one in a million. It's a long shot now, and it always has been." Each Saturday noon, as I left, I hoped that nothing terrible would happen. Eventually it did.

What a champion my boy was! Each week I felt as if I had let my prizefighter go into the ring with one of his gloved hands tied behind his back. Sometimes he was a skydiver dropped from a plane with a torn parachute. Other times, he was a deep-sea scuba diver with only half a tank of oxygen. Literally, all of Mike's emotions were gone. He could "feel" nothing, which was a true handicap for an actor. All actors draw on their past experiences to express emotions that create an illusion that interests or amuses their audience. Mike had to rely only on the memory of his emotions. He might well have been the greatest actor of all.

When Dr. Kim found out that Mike was back taking acting lessons, his response was, "The delusion might become the dream." I sat back and wondered why he didn't know that the dream had simply become delusional.

During the third lesson, all of my fears came true. Mike's acting teacher had asked all of the students in his class to "act" like a person with a mental illness. Many of these aspiring young actors tried to mimic a "split-personality" or "multiple personality disorder". Others "acted" hostile or threatening. Mike refused to participate in the exercise, and time had mercifully run out at the end of the lesson. He approached my car with a deeply troubled look.

"What's wrong, Mike?"

"Get me out of here, Mom."

"Do you want to stop at a fast food restaurant for lunch, Mike?"

"No, I'm not hungry," he said as he donned his sunglasses that blocked out the painful light. A beautiful, sunny winter day was not a gift for him. One of his medications, Cogentin, dilated his pupils and caused him severe pain in bright light.

"OK Mike, I'm going to go through McDonald's drive-through and get us some coffee. If you get hungry on the way home, we'll stop again." Mike remained silent for an hour.

Then he opened up and told me what had happened. "I wanted to say to all of them, Look at me! I am a schizophrenic. What do you see?" Mike made a bold attempt at crying but the tears would not come. Intellectually and strictly from memory, he understood but couldn't "feel" pain or joy. I didn't know what to say, except that they were stupid and uneducated people. Inside, I wrenched because I knew that there would be more of them to come. This was Mike's first official lesson on stigma.

With my stomach in my throat, I said, "Next week will be better, Mike."

Over the following two years, Mike occasionally had what we called "breakthrough symptoms". We never saw these symptoms as a relapse but responded to them quickly as a warning device. About every three to six months, Mike experienced mild somatic hallucinations such as sparkly lights in his field of vision, milder sensations from his forehead down his spine, and tingling sensations in his nose. Each time, we promptly reported the symptoms to Dr. Kim, who carefully increased Mike's Abilify just a little at a time. Each increase resulted in days of Mike's lying in bed as the medication kicked in and the milder drooling stopped. He described each increase by saying "The clamp tightened on my brain again." Unfortunately, one of these medication increases occurred right at the moment that someone from Hollywood had come to the agency to give further instructions during a weekend seminar. Mike only made it to the first lesson. I had to make excuses about a family reunion that Mike could not avoid, but this excuse was not well received by the owner of the agency. In spite of the fact that Mike had perfect attendance in the acting program previous to this, he fell from grace.

These weekly lessons were designed to prepare the acting students for a "once in a lifetime" opportunity for small-town kids to get in front of talent agents and managers from both the east and west coasts. Ironically, that opportunity came on July 29th, 2006, exactly one year after Mike's break from reality. For months, Michael's grandmother had spent hours each week helping him to select and then memorize three different one-minute monologues. One was serious, one humorous, and the last a commercial. These daily events developing themes and practicing together were planned between lunch and pinochle games.

Off we flew to New York City along with a large group of aspiring young actors and their parents. It was a five-day event, with early morning meetings and seminars for most of the day. Each student had several competitions with breakdowns according to their age. During the event, I spent a large amount of time with parents from our respective agency as well as with parents from other agencies located around the country. They were all quite lovely and claimed that they were simply there to allow their children to have the opportunity to compete in a safe environment. I agreed. Always, when the parents saw Mike, their responses were the same. "If your kid doesn't get a chance here, no one will. He's a handsome young man."

I had been friendly with the parents at Mike's school and agency but had kept them at arm's length. During the competition, I visited with them and spoke more freely. It became clear to me that they had previously thought I was a snob and that perhaps Mike was one as well.

On the last evening, we watched competitions from a large overhead projector and viewed the awards as we ate our final supper in New York City. I sat at a huge table that seated almost sixteen and visited with the other mothers from Mike's school and agency. It was the last night, and I was relieved that the tension was over. It was then that they opened up to me.

"We didn't know what to make of you, but you seem so down-to-earth now that we have had the chance to get to know you." I thanked them. "We really didn't understand your son. He's really an intellectual person, isn't he?"

"Yes, he is. Mike is a thinking person and very intelligent."

The other mothers had become quite close during the months of preparation for the event. I had stood at a watchful distance, interacting only when necessary. Now at the end, I was able to talk with them on a common level. Nothing had gone wrong! None of them knew that in between each class and competition Mike and I had gratefully slipped away to our hotel room, so that he might rest his mind. Sometimes he was very lucky and able to sleep for an hour. None of them had noticed when I discreetly handed Mike a plastic baggie that held his Cogentin to take mid-day.

"Your son is so handsome. Did he get any offers or awards? My child didn't."

"Yes, he got one offer. He also got an honorable mention for his commercial presentation."

Six months later, Mike and I flew to LA for an acting seminar and an audition in front of twenty agents and managers. We spent several days touring Hollywood and visited most of the famous sites. The day-long seminar took place in a rented facility. I dropped Mike off, knowing that he could still be a little vague, and went next door to a Mexican restaurant for lunch, hoping once again that nothing would go wrong. Many other parents were there, and we quickly became good short-term friends. At the appointed time that parents were allowed back for the parents' seminar, we all returned together. It was made expressly clear to all of us that no matter what the outcomes of the auditions were, if you want your child to succeed in Hollywood, you need to live here.

I had left on this voyage to the west coast worrying about two things: "What will happen if they actually want him? What will happen if they don't?" Either way, it was a losing proposition. The positive thing was that Mike had the chance and the ability to audition in a competitive environment. I viewed this whole experience as a miracle in itself.

On the plane ride home, I spoke to Michael candidly. "Mike, we can't move out here right now. I would love to send you out here, but you can't take care of yourself completely right now. Don't you agree? You still need a lot of support Mike. It's Dad's healthcare insurance that pays for your expensive medicine. We simply don't have any other options right now." With a heavy heart, I presented an honest sense of reality. "Mike, we are totally out of money. All of this has been quite expensive."

"I know Mom, but I will miss this."

Chapter 27 – Remission

The clinical description of remission is twofold: (1) Lessening of severity or abatement of symptoms. (2) The period during which symptoms abate or decrease. This description came directly from my *Taber's Cyclopedic Medical Dictionary* (1975), which I had saved from my nursing school days. In reviewing the meaning of these words, the definitions were still true. Nothing was said about a cure. "Lessening of severity" brought with it a partial sense of relief. "The period during which symptoms abate" brought a complete panic and dread. How long would Mike's remission last?

After one year of trial and error, with dosage adjustments of both Abilify and Cogentin, Michael had achieved 90% remission. The infrequent ghost of a "voice" might say to Mike, "Wait a minute." The sparkling stars in his field of vision and mild somatic "surges" in his nose or down his spine still occasionally happened. Mike had learned to live with them.

As many as two weeks went by with many "good days" in which Mike was engaging with friends and family and participating in routine activities. Then followed the bad days, when Mike's eyes looked haunted as he spent most of the day lying in bed, but unable to sleep. Some of this could have been attributed to his occasional inability to think clearly, as in putting ideas together that made sense. Some of it was simply depression. "Mother, how could this have happened to me? I had but one life, and this is what happened?" His friends remained true and loyal. They included him in all their activities, but they were moving forward in their own lives.

Well-meaning friends and family suggested that it would be good for Mike to get a part-time job. "Why is it that he can attend these acting classes but can't work a few hours a week?" I knew that Mike was a gentleman and put on a very good front, which confused them. But they didn't understand the truth. Background noises still occurred and exhausted him. The side effects of his drugs were disabling. He completely lacked energy, except for the brief spurts in which he pushed himself to the maximum. It would take two years and eight months to see any real improvement. Out of self-preservation and the lack of will or energy to educate the persistently obtuse, I avoided and dismissed those who didn't comprehend, sometimes quite harshly.

After one year into his disease, Mike was able to show us deep love and gratitude. This ability that he retained was a gift to us. "Thank you, Mom and Dad, for taking care of me," had become almost a daily assertion.

Mike's ability to read for a prolonged period of time and retain information was diminished. His tremendous mathematical skills were gone. Adding up a pinochle score was difficult. This was inconceivable to me as I remembered that Mike had tutored his roommates and friends in college. Mike said after one year, "I understood the language of mathematics." Could it be that the language part of his brain had been the most damaged?

Even after Mike's remission, on a bad day, he often asked, "Mom, if I should suddenly become psychotic again, will you help me out of this?" I listened to what he asked, contemplating his fear and urgency. Sadly, I knew first that I didn't have the courage to offend Almighty God. Second, I knew that it was wrong. I told Mike that treatments were rapidly advancing.

"You are the bravest man that I know, Mike."

"Why, Mom? Because I keep walking?"

"Yes, because you keep walking."

Mike had told me in elaborate detail how he had planned to commit suicide during the previous months. "Car in the garage, carbon monoxide from the exhaust system, delivered by a hose would do it." I came home from work each afternoon and looked for his car in the driveway. I wondered if he was still with me. I was always relieved to find that he was simply out driving and listening to his music as I quickly checked the garage. I unloaded my car from my day on the road and thought, "It didn't happen today, but I couldn't blame him if he left me on his own terms." This was no ordinary disease. It was a war. My boy had been captured, tortured, and was a POW. No one seemed to understand this.

My mother, who had lovingly raised her large family almost single-handedly as Dad worked long and unrelenting hours, once told me, "Children are only yours on loan. Do the very best you can to love, nurture, and fill them with good advice. Sooner or later, they will leave you." My parents were full of wisdom, which I thought of in the long and trying dark days.

Going back to remission and the period during which symptoms abate, we appreciated each and every moment when Mike was with us. The "loan" part of my mother's advice might have been far more significant for us than for others.

Chapter 28 – *2007*

The New Year rang in as usual at midnight, and we gratefully waved goodbye to 2006, another painful, unforgettable year. At the end of January, Mike was scheduled to compete in LA and we would ultimately have to decide that we could no longer go forward with long-distance auditions. We could no longer afford the expensive acting lessons that were given almost two hours away. Mike had demonstrated his bravery, strength, and perseverance, in spite of all odds. The new obstacles were money, insurance benefits, and Mike's ongoing need for a strong support system. He had continued to improve with each ninety-day interval, but it would take a full two years and eight months to see dramatic improvement. Gradually, his reading and mathematical skills returned, but his physical and mental stamina were still quite limited. He had pushed himself to compete in a world that even the healthy and lucky found difficult, exhausting all his available energies.

Mike needed more than video games and movies to occupy his time as Mark and I worked. His grandparents continued to include him in pinochle games and lunch each day, but he needed a purpose even if it seemed quite small in the minds of others. We would ask Mike if he didn't want to join a gym. This suggestion was met with a positive response from Mike, and he began to exercise three times a week.

"Mike, why don't you get a part-time job?" Mike tried to explain that he was not up to this task, but the kind suggestions became more forceful and insistent from family and friends.

"Mother, I have been lying in bed for most of the last two years. That is what it's taken to come this far." We understood the severity of his brain injury and asked others to let him get better at his own pace. Later we learned through our NAMI "Family to Family" lessons that most people who suffer an acute psychotic episode remain both physically and mentally exhausted for at least two years. The chemical assault that occurred to their brains caused damage that was just as real as a stroke or traumatic head injury. These lessons validated what we had already seen, but at the time we simply listened to Mike and allowed him to have control over his own recovery. We only knew three things we could do to reduce the chance of a relapse. The first was to be diligent and consistent in medication adherence. The second was to reduce stress. The third was to promptly report any symptoms that might arise, requiring medication adjustment to head off an acute exacerbation. Our knowledge was limited, but our instincts were good. *Give this kid some control over his life! Let him decide when he's ready for the next step.*

Spring arrived, and another ninety days passed with marked improvement. Kind suggestions that were made seemed more acceptable. "Mike," we said, "maybe you might consider going back to college. Why don't you try just one course this summer, to finish your degree? See how it goes." No pressure was put on him to succeed or even to pass the course. He enrolled in a speech course which seemed to fit in with his previous part-time acting classes. The result was a grade of B. This first step provided new confidence for Mike, and he took for two business courses in the fall which also resulted in B grades. Two thousand and seven proved to be a much better year.

The two-year anniversary of the saddest day of our lives was approaching, but Mark found a way to celebrate how far we had come since that dark day. We had acquired airline miles from the constant use of our MasterCard for business and personal expenses. A paid trip to the Pacific Northwest awaited us in August. Two years earlier, we had promised Mike on that fateful day that we would take him there on our next trip. The return trip to Seattle was anticipated with great joy! Our son was becoming healthy again, and he would come with us to watch the whales.

Our first day in Seattle was spent walking the waterfront, as we had done two years before, but this time Mike was with us. We toured an aquatic museum and ate supper at a lovely restaurant with a view of the Puget Sound. Each moment of the vacation was designed only to fulfill our needs and desires. The streets were just as hilly as I remembered as we visited the coffee and gift shops. Trudging uphill to tour the city had been somewhat difficult for me and humorous at once, with Mark pulling me by the hand and Mike pushing me from behind as we all laughed. Mike had only one true desire in touring Seattle. He wanted to see the Crocodile Café, where Kurt Cobain got his start. The building was as "grunge" as his band had been. Kurt had achieved huge fame and quick success, but later took his own life as a result of bipolar disorder.

It became immediately clear to me that there were hundreds of homeless people on the streets of Seattle. Why had I missed this on our last visit? This time I knew instantly that almost all of them were schizophrenic. I recognized their blazing eyes. I witnessed several men raising their arms to the sky in a "V." The street people who suffered from schizophrenia ruled the universe just as easily from the west coast as Mike had from the shores of Lake Erie. I observed their unusual gaits as they raised their legs up high while walking, never swinging their arms. Many of them begged for money or cigarettes. I was moved to great pity as I observed the symptoms of their disease, never once fearing them, but wondering why it had to be this way for them. Then, remembering the agony that Mike went through with the side effects of his medication, it became clear. These people preferred to live in a world full of delusions and hallucinations, rather than face the new anguish of their medications. I couldn't blame them, but wondered how they survived on a day-to-day basis. Did someone feed them? Was there any shelter or the opportunity for a shower? How did they keep warm at night? Did anybody even care?

I understood that it was also quite possible that many of them had "anosognosia." They might have had a decreased awareness of their disease, an innate inability to understand their diagnosis. I had read about this additional problem on the internet and in publications. If these poor people couldn't understand that they were sick, they also couldn't comprehend the need for medications that gave gruesome side effects. Once again, I felt contempt for the nursing staff in the psychiatric unit to which Mike had been admitted, on two occasions. Their staff's demeanor offended me deeply. Sometimes "the revolving doors" were not the fault of the patients who came and went with such frequency. Perhaps inadequate follow-up plans with support systems in place and the lack of a timely appointment with a psychiatrist before their medicine ran out caused them to lapse into this "other world." I felt deep compassion for all of these poor street people and thought, "It could have been Mike."

The next day, we drove up Route 5, heading north to the great city of Vancouver. We promptly checked into our hotel and embarked on a trip to Grouse Mountain. A skyline tram took us on a rail to the top of the mountain that overlooked the entire city of Vancouver. High and above the tall trees that resembled a forest on this mountain, the rail provided both a view and a destination. The surprises continued once we reached the top. There were many activities as well as wonderful views and walking trails on all sides.

"Restaurants", an outside zoo of sorts, featured a family of bears and a path exhibiting huge carvings of wildlife that were indigenous to the Pacific Northwest and Canadian Rockies; these were our delights. We spent several hours enjoying the views and attractions, had a late lunch, and suddenly felt the need for rest. In our minds, it was at least four hours later. Exhausted, we got in line to take the tram back to the ground level of the city. In the waiting line for the tram, we met a Canadian couple who were almost exactly our age. We introduced ourselves, struck up a quick conversation, and praised the beauty of their city. We discussed many topics, but one stood out in my mind quite clearly. I spoke to the wife and remarked that I had seen so many homeless people in Seattle. Her quick response was, "Well of course, they are almost all schizophrenic, you know. They exist here in Vancouver as well, and all up and down the Pacific Coast in the major cities."

"Why is that so?" I asked.

"The climate on the west coast is temperate." she responded quickly. "They can survive on the streets in the winter months." Together we rode the tram back down to the street level. Mike had not listened to our conversation as he viewed the wonders and beauty on the trip back.

"You would never believe that a person with schizophrenia was right beside you," I thought, as I smiled and bid them adieu.

The next day was devoted to a trip north to visit Whistler Mountain, the future site of the 2010 Winter Olympics. Our destination was quite breathtaking but competed with the trip there and back. We drove through the Canadian Rockies, a magnificent view in themselves, while looking west at the Pacific Ocean, home to spectacular mountains, nobly rising up from the depths of its deep blue water. I have, quite frankly, never seen a more beautiful sight in my life.

Our last day was spent in Anacorta, a small town north of Seattle on the Puget Sound, where we boarded a large vessel to go whale watching. We sat on the upper deck, warmed by sunshine and our newly purchased sweatshirts as we watched a herd of orcas swim behind our boat. The killer whales leapt almost like dolphins in our bubbling wake. It was a wonderful sight, only saddened by the thought that somehow, this time, with Mike at our side, the humpbacks were absent. Maybe such an exclusive experience only happens once in a lifetime. Perhaps it could happen for Mike, but we wouldn't be there.

We returned home with many happy memories of our wonderful adventure. We had a whole lot for which to be grateful. Our son was recovering. Somehow we had kept our family intact, one day at a time, as we muddled through the stresses that accompany a major and life-threatening illness. It was like we had an epiphany. We understood once again what we had always known. Nothing can replace the moment. One never knows what the next moment might hold.

Chapter 29 – Stigma and Ignorance

"Michael, you know that I've been writing a journal about our lives and your illness. I hope to get it published one day. I have already changed the names of persons, places, and things to protect the privacy of others. So far in my writing, I have kept only family names and our general location true and accurate. I can change all of them to fictitious names, including yours and mine. I can write my memoir using a pseudonym."

"No, Mom, keep our names as they are. The only way to combat the stigma is to tell the truth. All of the people that I care about already know. I want my picture on the cover of your book." Mike was absolutely fearless as we discussed my venture to chronicle what he had been through. In spite of his resolution, I feared that there might be serious consequences in the future.

"Do you want to read what I have written, Mike?"

"No, Mother, I lived it, but you were there. I'll read it when you get it published."

I worried about future employment opportunities along with future potential relationships with women. Then I thought that the only way to break the chain of ignorance and confusion regarding illnesses of the brain was to prove that people could get better and achieve their goals. Mike was indeed one of the luckier ones among those who developed this terrible illness, but I believe that with the newer medications and research, people afflicted with schizophrenia have a much better chance at leading a fuller life.

The ignorance factor was sometimes easier to deal with than the stigma factor, but not always. Friends, family, and neighbors learned from me that schizophrenia usually occurs at the end of puberty and the onset of adulthood. It is during this period that the final "pruning" of neurons (nerve cells of the brain) occurs. One theory is that an environmental "insult" such as an infection during the middle trimester of pregnancy may later result in a problem with this final development of the brain. Difficult births and retroviruses are also under scrutiny as contributing factors to the development of the disease, along with a genetic predisposition or vulnerability.

Latent (dormant) viruses are suspect. We already know that the Varicella-zoster virus causes chickenpox, and after years of dormancy in the body can flare up again and cause "shingles," a painful condition in which the virus attacks nerves along the face or back. Victims of the polio virus, who had already survived paralysis and iron lungs to help them breathe in their youths, sadly develop a milder form of the disease known as "post-polio syndrome," thirty years later.

Another theory is that schizophrenia is simply a bad consequence of evolution, as the left side and right side of the brain have become better adapted to communicate with each other.

The human brain is such a complicated organ with so many functions! Not only is it the seat of consciousness, thought, memory, reason, judgment, and emotion, but a living, breathing computer that communicates with all other organs in the body. The brain is indeed the "Master Organ," and to some degree "bosses" other organs around! When cognition, simply one function of the brain, becomes impaired, the uneducated suspect that stress is the culprit! This rationale has caused me to feel deep discomfort and frustration. "Stress" is a human condition, in response to an imperfect world, but certainly not all people who experience stress develop schizophrenia.

The stigma factor was met with my complete contempt and total lack of interest in educating people who were clearly not highly evolved in matters of humanity. Occasionally I heard, first-hand or second-hand, labels that people applied to Mike's brain disease: "crazy" or "nuts." We live in a small town. I have always known that "telling one person something meant telling them all." I thought, *They must all know now and who cares? We have already looked into the gaping doors of Hell.*

My parents had told me long ago, "If at the end of your life, you can count five good friends on the fingers of one hand, you are lucky." As always, they were right with their "wisdoms" on life. For years, strong winds would blow and shake out the fruit from the trees. The fruit that remained were friends who simply listened. Like my brother Mike, they offered no opinions or unsolicited advice. With my frustration over peoples' ignorance, I also learned how many good people genuinely cared about me. These were my customers and people at the furniture factory I represented. Many had been praying for our family for months. Each person had put us on their own church's prayer list. There must have been thousands of people praying for Mike.

I was in my fifties and understood that a lot of ignorant people walk this earth among us. The stigma of Mike's disease was inconsequential to me until it caused Mike pain. Then I took it quite personally and was outraged. Mike's "first official lesson on stigma" at his acting school, when his teacher had asked the students to "act" like a person with a mental illness, was mild compared to what Mike would face again, alone.

David, Mike's oldest best friend, had recently purchased a house and hosted a Halloween party. Mike was invited to spend the night and join in the festivities. There were a number of guests Mike had known previously, but a few that he had never met. A small group of guests had become quite intoxicated by midnight; among them was a young woman who was majoring in psychology at the local university. Apparently, she was quite colorful as she described her clinical experiences at the local hospital and described all the "dangerous" schizophrenics. Her stories were followed by a number of embarrassing jokes delivered by her drunken companions.

Michael kept his composure. He asked the party of four people, "Do you think that in any everyday situation, that you might meet a schizophrenic on the street?" The drunken woman thought it was certainly possible. Mike continued, "Do you think that if you go into a grocery or department store, the person checking you out might have schizophrenia?"

"Well, maybe."

"Do you think that there might be a schizophrenic in one of your college classes?"

"It could happen, but it's unlikely."

"Do you think that there just might be one here in this room, right in front of you?"

"I doubt that."

"Well, I just want to announce that you're looking at one, and I don't find any of this funny."

The foursome tried to apologize as Michael left quite abruptly. Then David threw them out as they attempted to make excuses for their boorish behavior.

Michael immediately left, drove home, and awakened Mark and me at 2:00 in the morning. We put our heads down to cry as we heard the story, but indignantly said, "Mike, you did the right thing to leave and come home."

"It was brave of you to speak up, Mike," his father said through tears.

"This was nothing less than stupidity, Mike. Unfortunately, there will be more stupid people. We can't stop that," I said with painful resignation.

Mike's emotions were coming back because he was able to have a good and cleansing cry. We had one with him.

Chapter 30 – Education and Hope

The single best decision that Mark and I have ever made was to become involved in our small NAMI (National Alliance on Mental Illness) support group. NAMI is a nonprofit, grassroots, self-help organization for people with mental illnesses and their families. With 210,000 members nationwide, NAMI is dedicated to the eradication of mental illnesses and provides a strong voice to our mental health system and government as advocates for people with brain disorders. Our small group met for twelve weeks, studying, sharing, and supporting each other, during our "Family to Family" program. We met some of the finest people we had ever known in our lives and we continue to meet once a month to share information, support, and love.

They say misery loves company, and some of this is true, but that is not the mission of our small group. We actually want to change things. Each of my NAMI mothers and fathers has a different agenda on how they plan to accomplish their goals, and all of them are active in their own way. We are all "soft," but "fighters" at the same time. We share newspaper and magazine articles along with books we have read. I reported to our group the increasing number of newscasters and politicians who had been "poetically" speaking about our "schizophrenic government" and how misleading this terminology was to the general public. "What is the meaning – Crazy? Split Personality? Either way, we all know that this isn't good reporting or campaigning."

Some of my friends are active in the legal system and devote their time to educating local law officers about how to deal with a crisis. Simple procedures to de-escalate a situation are taught along with basic education on mental illnesses. Too often, people with severe mental illnesses have been shot and killed when uncomplicated techniques could have brought a quiet resolution.

As NAMI members, we all know that the rate of violent crimes that occurs with people suffering from schizophrenia who are properly medicated is exactly the same as within the general population. Yet the media never fails to emphasize when some bizarre crime involves a person with a mental illness.

Can a person who suffers from schizophrenia, or any other severe mental illness, become aggressive or even violent in their confusion? My answer to that question is, certainly. So can the elderly suffering from dementia, patients in severe pain, or those recovering from anesthesia. My years in nursing had brought many experiences in dealing with patients who were temporarily or permanently confused. Nurses around the world, who care for the confused, have been slapped, punched, kicked, and bitten. Yet, it's the sacred secret, never mentioned to the patient's family or broadcast on the news. Confusion is simply a period of time in which a person doesn't have complete control over their faculties.

With proper education in place for parents, young adults, educators, and other professionals, early diagnosis, vigorous treatment, and, more importantly, conscientious follow-up care could potentially prevent violent crimes before they occur. The term "conscientious follow-up care" reminds me that not everyone who has a "first psychotic episode" has an "Uncle Mike" to take care of him/her during the earliest days, when the most urgent needs must be met. I am also reminded that not every parent has a "Brother Jim" to handle employment respon-sibilities at the most critical time. Just as our government must face the needs of the elderly and the mentally or physically handicapped, we must face the needs of our citizens who suffer from organic brain diseases. Medical doctors should use their expertise and wisdom to custom-design the course of treatment for people suffering from brain diseases, omitting the "assistance" of uneducated bureaucrats deciding which drugs are approved due to cost, without regard to efficacy. But first we must actually believe that people with schizophrenia can and will recover.

Each month, our NAMI support group has a round table, with parents reporting their concerns or triumphs involving their children. We all live in hope. My friends know that writing is on my agenda. While my writing has been something of a cathartic experience, that wasn't my singular goal. When my memoir is published, if only people that "already know" read it, my efforts would be nothing more than "preaching to the choir". My primary goal is to reach the parents of recently diagnosed children and to give them hope, as they witness the same sad events occurring in their own beloved child. My secondary goals are equally ambitious but lofty. Is it possible to reach parents of mentally well children and let them walk in my shoes for just a short time? Perhaps these parents might become advocates for people who develop mental illnesses. Possibly others could identify the early warning symptoms and somehow head off the catastrophe early on, with small doses of medication. Could I change the heart of one callous nurse and make him/her understand that each patient he/she cares for is "someone's child." My very first thought of wisdom regarding mental illness was that if this could happen to Mike, it could happen to anyone.

Schizophrenia is a tragic disease that approaches secretively and insidiously. It arrives just like a thief in the night. Thieves don't openly announce themselves before they come to steal what you treasure most in life. Could it happen to your child?

Chapter 31 – Keeping Good Company

After Mike's illness, I searched the Internet and books that told about famous people who had developed schizophrenia. I was surprised to find that we were keeping very good company. My best resource *Surviving Schizophrenia*, by Dr. E. Fuller Torrey, M.D., names a number of people. Dr. Torrey has written that poet Robert Frost, had an aunt, a son, and perhaps a daughter who developed the disease. Albert Einstein's son, daughters of Victor Hugo, Bertrand Russell, and James Joyce were also victims of schizophrenia. French writer Antonin Artaud, American painter Ralph Blakelock, English composer and poet Ivor Gurney, American mathematician John Nash, and Russian dancer Vaslov Nijinsky are cited as creative individuals who suffered from the disease.

The son of Kurt Vonnegut, the famous bestselling novelist, developed schizophrenia. Vonnegut's son survived the illness and later became an author himself as well as a pediatrician. Actor Alan Alda, famous for his key role in *M*A*S*H* (1972-1982) as well as many other highly acclaimed films, wrote a book about his mother, who suffered from schizophrenia.

Schizophrenia For Dummies , written by Jerome Levine, M.D. and Irene S. Levine, PhD, provided names of other famous people who were afflicted: Lionel Aldridge (of the Green Bay Packers), Syd Barrett (founding member of Pink Floyd), Jim Gordon (drummer for Derek and the Dominoes), Peter Green, (guitarist and founder of Fleetwood Mac), Tom Harrell (jazz musician), Jack Kerouac (poet), Mary Todd Lincoln (First Lady), and Brian Wilson (bass player and singer for the Beach Boys).

There were many other famous people throughout history who most likely developed the disease. No modern-day psychiatrists were available to put a name to their disorder. Only their symptoms remain in the chronicles of history, blatantly describing their brain disease.

As I perused this interesting information, I understood that while Mike was certainly good-looking and very intelligent, he wasn't a genius. We were nothing more than a hard-working middle class family trying to stay ahead of the next bill or catastrophe to come. We weren't famous or extraordinary people. Why then did I feel so compelled to write about Mike's tribulations? Why was it so easy to tell the truth about what had happened to him? He was getting better. Why not hide the whole thing and go on with our lives? Why disclose everything and potentially put our only child at risk for future stigma and prejudice? We were just ordinary people who happened to have a positive outcome from this dreadful disease. That must have been the compelling reason.

Chapter 32– Proud Parents

Evan, who was Michael's best friend and college roommate, was getting married to Alissa in early November 2008, and he chose Mike to be his best man. The church was decorated beautifully in autumn-colored flowers as traditional wedding music played. Mark and I stood just outside the door, looking fondly and with admiration at our handsome son as he waited calmly, then attentively ushered guests to their pews. I snapped a picture of him and the other groomsmen, who were also Mike's and Evan's high school buddies. They all looked so young and handsome in their dashing brown tuxedos.

Mike approached and asked to escort us to a pew. "Michael, you look like a million bucks!"

"Thanks, Mom. I have quite a few more duties to perform before I can really relax. I want to do a good job as best man for Evan and Alissa." In the traditional manner, Mark followed as I was escorted down the aisle by our son. Mike smiled at me gallantly as I held onto his arm and kissed me as we reached our destination on the groom's side of the church. Mike and his father patted each other on the back appropriately, in father-son affirmation and affection.

Mark and I sat in our pew, waiting for the ceremony to begin. We admired the young men Mike had known since his youth complete their duties as ushers. The bride entered on the arm of her father, looking radiantly beautiful as she approached the altar. It was one of the loveliest weddings we had ever attended. The wedding ceremony was a Catholic Mass. Alissa's uncle, a deacon of the church, delivered the sermon and brought beautiful Polish influences and Polish-language sayings into the theme of this union.

As the newly-wed couple was announced by the priest to the world, with loud clapping from the audience, they proceeded down the aisle. I snapped my camera quickly. What a lovely young couple they were! What confidence we felt in this new marriage! We watched our son escort the maid of honor and snapped his picture along with many others as the wedding party proceeded from the church.

The reception was second only in good taste to the ceremony itself. The traditions, food, and entertainment echoed the real souls of the newly united couple. Their honest desire to share their happiness and celebration with family and friends had been paramount in planning of the event. The cake was cut and then the toasting began.

Ray, the disc jockey, also served as master of ceremonies. He introduced the wedding party members as they offered their toasts to the new couple. Alissa's bridesmaids, who were her sisters, gave very emotional, loving speeches and toasts honoring the bride and groom. The bridesmaids were saying goodbye to their sister but welcoming a wonderful brother-in-law. Then it was time for the best men to give toasts, and there were two of them. Robert went first and delivered a heart-warming monologue filled with emotion for the newlyweds. Then Mike was up.

"Are you ready, Mike?" Ray asked over the microphone.

"I was born ready, Ray!" Mike cheerfully retorted. Six weeks earlier, he had artfully and carefully crafted twelve sentences to be delivered at this moment. I had been surprised at his ability to write so succinctly. His first points involved good-natured humor about their college days. Some were designed to be thoughtful and sensitive about Evan's kind nature. The last described accurately why Evan and Alissa were so well suited for each other and made each other complete. Mike was met with a loud round of applause. It was an excellent toast, and Mike had delivered it well.

"That's our boy!" Mark and I whispered to each other. I thought that Mike's acting lessons in 2006 and his college speech class in 2007 had really paid off. Michael had spoken directly into the microphone as he addressed over 300 people. His voice was well modulated, and his toast had not been delivered too quickly. He had waited for appropriate responses to each sentence, whether they might be laughter or pause for thought. He had saved the best and closing statements for the end as he delivered his toast to the new couple.

Finally Mike was done with his major responsibilities. After supper, he approached our table and described his relief to Mark and me. "I was really nervous. There are over 300 people in this room! Could you see my hand shaking as I held my notes?"

"No, we couldn't, Mike. You did a great job delivering your toast. We were proud of you!"

"Mother, would you like to dance?" Mike asked as the music started. It was a great song and after this slow dance was over, his father stepped in for the next.

Mike later approached me and asked, "Mom, do you want to go outside and have a smoke with me?"

"Yes, I am sure ready." We smoked our cigarettes outside the banquet hall in the cold and discussed the success of the entire day. "This was a wonderful wedding, Mike. You certainly did your part to help make it go well." We reentered the hall and ran into Mike's friend's father, who is a doctor.

"Mike, how is it going with you? Are you still pursuing acting?" Dr. Richards asked.

"Right now, I'm finishing my degree in business," Mike replied, "so that I'll have a job that pays well with benefits, but I haven't forgotten my dream, Dr. Richards. I'd like to try it again, but I want to be able to support myself in the meantime."

"That's smart, Mike. It's nice to see you again." I wondered if Dr. Richards "knew."

Evan, the groom, pulled me out of my seat twice to dance with me. What a nice boy! Both times I kept my focus on him and Alissa. "This is such a beautiful wedding, Evan. I am so happy for you and Alissa!" Anthony, a groomsman and long-term friend of both Evan and Mike, also dragged me from my seat twice to dance. I thought it was quite chivalrous for Anthony to dance with an old lady in the crowd. I called him by his old nick-name, "Tony, Mike looks good; don't you think?"

"Yes," he replied, "Mike's doing great because you and Mike's dad were both there for him."

"Thank you," I said with a smile. But what I really thought was that we were incredibly lucky.

Mike was attending college at a local state university, taking extremely challenging courses in business with an emphasis on computers. Aside from his remarkably good looks, manners, sweet disposition, and heritage, one thing set him apart from many other young people. Michael was a survivor of schizophrenia. He had been to places that no one wants to visit, and he returned to this very ordinary world intact.

Chapter 33 – Conclusion

What an odd word 'conclusion' is! It means the end of a story, the completion and summing up of my memoir that can't be accomplished, because there is no end. Michael Dunham is a work in progress that can't yet be defined, except by his courage.

It must have been three years into Mike's disease when I had asked him to describe his level of recovery from schizophrenia. I was happily surprised by most of his answers.

"Mom, my intellectual abilities are all back, but I still have trouble reading for long periods of time and comprehending what I have read. Sometimes paying attention for long periods of time is a problem too, but I have learned how to compensate by taking notes and reviewing study materials in my college classes."

"Mike, what about your ability to feel emotions?"

"Mother, I only have about 50% of my emotions back."

"What is that like, Mike?"

"Ma, it's like someone cut off both of my legs. I can't feel them but I can still walk."

Mike's incredible gift of speaking in colorful and descriptive metaphors had been restored. It was at this moment that I had my second thought of wisdom regarding mental illness: *This is simply another kind of disability.* I believed at this turning point that Mike could do almost anything if he simply put his mind to it. Yet, a couple years later, his answer to my question about his ability to feel emotions was quite different.

"Ma, it's been so long since I had my break. I can't accurately describe exactly how much of my emotions are back. I can only tell you that I'm as good as I can remember."

Through the last few years, I have attended a number of educational programs along with my NAMI mothers and friends. I have learned that there are medical doctors, psychologists, nurses, CPAs, teachers, mailmen, college professors, lawyers, high ranking military officials, and other functioning people who are survivors of schizophrenia. For some, it took years to tell the truth about their struggles with brain diseases and the torture of their medications. Still, other people can't tell for fear of losing their jobs despite of the fact that they function quite well. Quiet and heroic survivors of brain diseases walk among us. Often we don't know who they are, because they can't tell us. The truth might hurt their chance of survival in our uninformed and competitive world.

Mike continued to complete courses, resulting in a bachelor's degree in the school of business at a local state university. Mike divulged his schizophrenia to only a few of his professors, and only when his energies were compromised. Sometimes the period allowed to take a test was insufficient for him to accomplish the reading.

"Have you gone to Student Services to get extra help?" his professors asked.

"No," Mike responded, "I want to do this on my own."

In May 2010, Mark and I sat in a huge auditorium, surrounded by proud parents who "expected it to turn out this way" as we watched our son, in cap and gown, receive his diploma. My husband leaned his leg against mine in an intimate moment that only people who have been married for a very long time can understand. "Susie, are you tearing up? I am."

"Mark, I've been crying since the start."

"Susie, we couldn't help him on this one. He did this all on his own."

Epilogue

It must have been two years into Mike's illness when I picked up and skimmed a newspaper offered on the counter of one of my furniture dealer's stores. I was waiting to see the buyer and amused myself by reading the articles. One in particular caught my attention. The column was clearly run each month and devoted to health care issues. This time the subject was stigma as related to mental illnesses. I quickly tucked the "free" newspaper into my binder.

Usually, when I got home, after making sure that things were "all right", I quickly got on to my faxes and emails and solved the problems of the day. But that afternoon I responded by email to the registered nurse who had written the article. It had been written so well that I felt compelled to contact her. As a result, we became email "pen pals" as well as NAMI members.

My trust in her became so complete that I felt comfortable sending her my unedited manuscript to read. Her comments were not only thorough but also kind. Eventually, we spoke to each other on the phone.

"Susie, why don't you come to our NAMI Walk? You might reach people who would be interested in your book." While her thoughtful suggestion was welcome, promoting the book wasn't my motive in attending. By nature I am an inquisitive and social being. What are these "NAMI Walks" all about?

One week before Mike's graduation from college, I travelled to a larger community to try to understand how the events that I had read about actually happened. What an interesting experience I had! NAMI Walks are designed to increase social awareness about mental illnesses and to raise money to educate the public. There must have been at least two hundred people in attendance, from all walks of life. The afflicted, family members, business people, social workers, other professionals, and nuns were involved in the fundraiser. As in the past when attending conventions or seminars, I had noticed determining who had a brain disease and who didn't was sometimes difficult. It was only my trained eye, as a former nurse, that allowed me to identify the long-term residual side effects of antipsychotics in this population.

I mingled with the crowd and attempted to join in their conversations. Coffee, hot chocolate, and soft drinks were available along with pastries and pizza for participants. All snacks and refreshments had been donated by local businesses.

I ventured toward the three elderly nuns who were dressed in sweat-suits and walking shoes, and approached the most smiling of the three.

"Sister, thank you for participating in this event, which is so important," I said. "My only child got schizophrenia in 2005. He suffered terribly, Sister, but he has recovered. He's the bravest person that I know. Next week he will graduate from college!" With her beautiful, aged, crippled, and arthritic hand, she pulled me close to her face.

"My dear," she said, with the compassionate eyes and a tender voice, "that's wonderful, but you had to be strong too!" I almost choked upon her inordinate praise as I remembered all of my frailties. Quickly, I recoiled from her but pointed to the heavens.

"I got a lot of help, Sister."

I was introduced by my NAMI pen pal to a number of people but made my own way through the crowd. I introduced myself to a lady who appeared to be about sixty-five years old. Her name badge announced that she was a case-worker in another community. After describing Michael's suffering and my venture to write about his recovery, I was taken completely off-guard by a warm bear-hug and a kiss on the cheek.

"Good for you," she said, "for telling the truth. Recovery is possible and happens more often than you might believe."

"You know, I think that it just takes everything you have, to help someone get well," was my response.

"And more," she added.

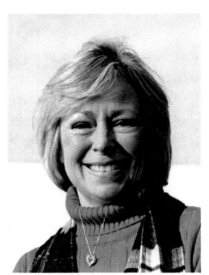

About the Author

Where did you grow up?

Born in Cleveland, the "later in life," unexpected seventh child of eight, I spent my pre-school years living above my father's furniture store. "Joe Ralph Furniture" was a profitable but mostly a family operation, with my mother the bookkeeper and my older siblings doing the manual labor. Each summer, my mother loaded up her tribe of children to spend three glorious months in a cement block cottage on the shores of Lake Erie. There my older siblings had jobs working for our grandmother at "Saylor's Place", a restaurant that specialized in smoked ribs, hosting a casual atmosphere along with white-tablecloth dining. My grandmother also owned a small marina and motel which required a teenage work force, easily fulfilled by my six older siblings. Eventually we left the big city and moved to Port Clinton, Ohio, a small community located on Lake Erie, where my father became as a manufacturer's sales rep in the furniture industry. I grew up in a "turn of the century" house that was spacious enough to house our large family, where faith, family unity, and a strong work ethic were the absolute rules.

Why are you uniquely qualified to write this book

In 1976, I graduated from Sandusky School of Practical Nursing and enjoyed a variety of experiences performing my own "art" in nursing. Three years in a hospital environment, five years in a nursing home setting and two in private duty nursing provided a wealth of information about the human spirit. I learned that patients are people, not diagnoses! During my brief tenure in nursing, I heard many times that the "fractured femur" in Room 108 wasn't comfortable on his current pain medication. Sometimes, the "congestive heart" in Room 110 needed increased diuretic because their urinary output wasn't sufficient to match their intake of fluids. Or, it was the "old schizophrenic" in Room 102 whose blood pressure was up. In report, none of them had names — just health problems that needed to be resolved. For many years, I cared for "people" who had a primary diagnosis of schizophrenia and suffered other health problems. Somehow, in my youth, I understood the sadness of their brain disorder. Just at the moment of final maturity, their lives had been stolen. They were left behind, not allowed to go forward to reap the benefits of their hard work. Some had been confined to mental institutions for as long as fifty years. I understood that for them, "life really wasn't fair."

Why did you write this book?

At first my writing was nothing more than journaling, writing short vignettes out of pain and catharsis. As time went on, I believed I had actually started writing a book. In the beginning, I was unsure whether the ending would be one of tragedy or triumph. I simply knew I was compelled to tell our story. I wanted to put a beautiful face that belonged to a brave, kind spirit on a tragic, horrific disease. I hoped that by introducing Michael as a healthy "all-American" kid, a real person, that anyone could identify him with their own child. Perhaps I could separate his lovely being from an unfortunate diagnosis — a label — and cause others to understand that he was a person suffering from schizophrenia, and not a schizophrenic. My very first thought of wisdom on mental illnesses was: *If this could happen to Michael, it could happen to anyone.* I understood that once you tell the truth, you can't "un-tell" it, and I realized that there was indeed risk involved. But my brave son Michael encouraged me to go forward. My greatest aspiration became reaching the parents of children who had been recently diagnosed, in their early, painful mourning period. I wanted these parents to believe that no matter what they were witnessing and no matter what pain their child was enduring, recovery was possible.

What do you think readers will get out of it?

I humbly acknowledge that medications and possible outcomes have improved over the last twenty years since I left nursing. Yet, there is so much room for improvement! As American citizens, we must take responsibility for education about mental illnesses, support the needs of people with brain diseases, and provide opportunities for them not only to barely survive—but thrive! But first we must actually believe that they can get better and be productive citizens. My efforts weren't focused only on telling our personal story but to dispel the myths surrounding schizophrenia. Schizophrenia is a non-discriminating medical disease that remains poorly understood, feared, and stigmatized due to a lack of proper information. Scientists are currently investigating brain activity on a cellular level, questioning whether the disease is simply a chemical imbalance or a lack of elasticity in brain neurons. It is my belief that standards must be universally set and met in our mental healthcare system, which is apparently broken. I also understand from my years in nursing that it is critical for nurses to maintain an emotional distance in the face of tragedy for their own survival.

But it is also equally important for psychiatric nurses to arm themselves with reliable sources of information and try to identify with the suffering involved in mental illness, helping them to provide compassion and advocacy. For a nurse to immediately presume that all of his/her efforts are for naught becomes a self-fulfilling prophesy. It might be a better idea for hospitals to offer in-service credit hours devoted to spending time with "real people" suffering from mental illnesses and their families as they attempt to meet the challenges of our current mental health care system. A good place to start would be in psychiatric wards, with attending nurses required to attend NAMI "Family to Family" classes. Better discharge resources designed to empower patients and their caregivers along with better follow-up plans of care would provide improved long-term outcomes. *Michael's recovery prompted my second thought of wisdom on mental illness. This is simply a different kind of disability.*

What will you do next in your life?

Education about mental illnesses and possible causes must start with the very young and continue throughout their school years. I would love to write an illustrated book designed for very young children that is age-appropriate, with simple and easy-to-understand words and terms. Because the myths about schizophrenia have persisted for such so long, perhaps it might be a worthy endeavor to start with our babies before they are influenced by outdated and incorrect dogma.

Appendix A - Recommended Reading

Green, M. (2001). *schizophrenia revealed: from neurons to social interactions.* New York: Norton

In easily understandable scientific terms, Dr. Green explores brain development, cellular activity, and genetics as related to schizophrenia. Clearly recognizing the personal costs of the disease, he offers hope as we look to the near future with fresh approaches in research and new medications.

Greenberg, M. (2008). *Hurry down sunshine.* New York: Other Press

Courageously honest, Michael Greenberg describes his daughter's sudden onset of psychosis due to bi-polar disease, subsequent hospitalization, and the impact her disease had on his family.

Hayes, L. (2009). *Mental illness and your town: 37 ways for communities to help and heal.* Ann Arbor: Loving Healing Press

Since 1930, in its original red and white plaid cover, *Better Homes and Gardens Cook Book* has provided easy and reliable recipes that allowed us to nourish our families. Larry Hayes' 37 proven "recipes" to empower people suffering from brain diseases are equally dependable and could easily be implemented in any community with great success. He calls to action all members of communities, stressing education, involvement, and our responsibility to provide opportunities for people who suffer from mental illnesses to thrive, instead of barely surviving.

Levine, J. & Levine, S. (2009). *Schizophrenia for dummies.* Hoboken: Wiley

Easy-to-read and user-friendly, this book offers information, resources and many helpful tips.

Schiller, L. & Bennett, A. (1996). *The quiet room: A journey out of the torment of madness.* New York: Warner Books

Bravely written, Lori Schiller recounts the onset of her frightening auditory symptoms as a teenager, recurrent hospital-izations, self-medication with cocaine, and ultimate recovery with the medication clozapine.

Steele, K. & Berman, C. (2001). *The day the voices stopped.* New York: Basic Books

Ken Steele's legacy lives on with the publication he started, *New York City Voices.* From the age of fourteen and lasting for thirty-two years, he lived a tragic life, impoverished and victim-ized as a result of a dysfunctional mental health system. When his symptoms were miraculously relieved by the medication risperidone, he became an activist and advocate for people living with severe mental illnesses.

Temes, R. (2002). *Getting your life back together when you have schizophrenia.* Oakland: New Harbinger Publications

Incredibly sensitive, helpful, and hopeful as well as easy to read and understand, Dr. Temes has written a primer for people suffering from schizophrenia and their families.

Torrey, E. (2006). *Surviving schizophrenia: A manual for families, patients and providers.* New York: HarperCollins

Now in its fifth edition, widely read throughout the world, Dr. E. Fuller Torrey's book remains the most comprehensive and authoritative work available on schizophrenia.

Tracey, P. (2008). *Stalking irish madness: Searching for the roots of my family's schizophrenia.* New York: Bantam Dell

This literary classic on schizophrenia probes into history, genetics, and environmental factors that may have impacted the prevalence of the disease in Ireland. Patrick Tracey tells the story of his pilgrimage to Ireland to uncover the roots of schizophrenia in his family. Heaped with sensitivity, compassion, and Irish lore, this book is a page-turner.

Wagner, P. & Spiro, C. (2006). *Divided minds: Twin sisters and their journey through schizophrenia.* New York: St. Martin's Press

Born with exactly the same genes, brought up in exactly the same environment, highly intelligent identical twin sisters' lives take different paths. "Pammy" develops schizophrenia, and "Lynnie" goes on to become a psychiatrist. This compelling story of sisterly love leads one to ask, *What are the real origins of schizophrenia?*

Appendix B - Internet Resources

(In alphabetical order)

www.nami.org

The website for the National Alliance on Mental Illness (NAMI), a non-profit, grassroots, self-help, support, and advocacy organization of consumers, families, and friends of people with severe mental illnesses, provides a wealth of information.

www.narsad.org

The National Alliance for Research on Schizophrenia and Affective Disorders raises money from donors around the world and invests 100% of all donations directly to research.

www.nimh.nih.gov

Federally funded, the National Institute of Mental Health's (NIMH) mission is to transform the understanding of mental illness through basic and clinical research, paving the way for prevention, recovery, and cure.

http://gauss.nimh.nih.gov/sibstudy/

Sponsored by the National Institute of Mental Health, this website invites you to participate in genetic studies. My husband, son, and I participated in a "Family Trio Study" which was incredibly easy to do. Simple questionnaires, phone interviews, and blood draws performed in our family doctor's office were all that were necessary. Volunteers are not given the results of the tests, but this easy and altruistic donation to science will benefit others as we search for the causes of schizophrenia. As in any other scientific study, with more people participating, the conclusions will be more accurate. All information is strictly confidential and ultimately your family will only be known by a "case number." What a great way to help science!

www.schizophrenia.com

Listed under "Favorites" on my computer, this website is a leading non-profit web community dedicated to providing high quality information, support, and education to family members, caregivers, and individuals whose lives have been impacted by schizophrenia.

www.szmagazine.com

The official website for *SZ Magazine* includes a sampling of stories from the quarterly periodical which I highly recommend. *SZ Magazine* was created in 1994 by Bill MacPhee, a survivor of schizophrenia. He envisioned a magazine that could reach out and help those affected by schizophrenia. Easy to read, filled with professional content, personal stories, and helpful information, *SZ Magazine* is a "must-read" for people living with schizophrenia, their caregivers, and medical professionals.

Index

LaVergne, TN USA
12 January 2011
212125LV00001B/71/P

The Reflections of America Series

This series highlights autobiography, fiction, and poetry which express the quest to discover one's context within modern society.

- *Tales of Addiction: and Inspiration for Recovery* by Barbara Sinor, PhD
- *Saffron Dreams* by Shaila Abdullah
- *Confessions of a Trauma Junkie : My life as a Nurse Paramedic* by Sherry Jones Mayo
- *Love Each Day : Live each day so you would want to live it again* by Gail Bernice Holland
- *My Dirty Little Secrets: Steroids, Alcohol, and God -- The Tony Mandarich Story*
- *The Stories of Devil-Girl* by Anya Achtenberg
- *How to Write a Suicide Note: serial essays that saved a woman's life* by Sherry Quan Lee
- *Chinese Blackbird* by Sherry Quan Lee

"Literature that is not the breath of contemporary society, that dares not transmit the pains and fears of that society, that does not warn in time against threatening moral and social dangers--such literature does not deserve the name of literature; it is only a façade. Such literature loses the confidence of its own people, and its published works are used as wastepaper instead of being read."

-Aleksandr Solzhenitsyn (1918-2008